Protein-Energy Malnutrition and Intellectual Abilities

Communications 5

AFRIKA-STUDIECENTRUM · LEIDEN

JAN HOORWEG

Protein-Energy Malnutrition and Intellectual Abilities

A study of teen-age Ugandan children

MOUTON · THE HAGUE · PARIS

Publications in collaboration with the Afrika-Studiecentrum, Leiden:*

Communications

1. M.L. Daneel: The God of the Matopo Hills. An Essay on the Mwari Cult in Rhodesia. 1970
2. M.L. Daneel: Zionism and Faith-Healing in Rhodesia. Aspects of African Independent Churches. 1970
3. P.M. van Hekken & H.U.E. Thoden van Velzen: Land Scarcity and Rural Inequality in Tanzania. Some Case Studies from Rungwe District. 1972
4. Robert Buijtenhuijs: Mau Mau: Twenty Years After. The Myth and the Survivors. 1973
5. Jan Hoorweg: Protein-Energy Malnutrition and Intellectual Abilities. 1976

Change and Continuity in Africa

1. Robert Buijtenhuijs: Le Mouvement "Mau-Mau". Une révolte paysanne et anti-coloniale en Afrique noire. 1971
2. M.L. Daneel: Old and New in Southern Shona Independent Churches. Volume I: Background and Rise of the Major Movements. 1971
3. Network Analyses: Studies in Human Interaction. Edited by Jeremy Boissevain and J. Clyde Mitchell. 1973
4. M.L. Daneel: Old and New in Southern Shona Independent Churches. Volume II: Church Growth. Causative Factors and Recruitment Techniques. 1973
5. J.F. Holleman: Issues in African Law. 1974
6. H.L. van der Laan: The Lebanese Traders in Sierra Leone. 1975
7. B.E. Harrell-Bond: Modern Marriage in Sierra Leone. A Study of the professional group. 1975

* *The Afrika-studiecentrum cannot in any way be held responsible for the views or opinions expressed in these books.*

Cover-design by Jurriaan Schrofer
ISBN: 90 279 7752 6

Printed in the Netherlands

to Puck

Acknowledgements

At various times during the course of the research reported in this monograph I have been associated with the Kampala Child Nutrition Unit of the Medical Research Council, the Makerere Institute of Social Research, the Social Psychology Departments of Makerere University and Leiden University, and the African Studies Centre at Leiden. I want to thank the directors and former directors of these institutes and departments, in particular Dr. R. Whitehead, Prof. Dr. P. Rigby, Prof. Dr. M. Segall, and Drs. G. Grootenhuis, for the confidence they have placed in me and the freedom they have allowed me.

I am above all indebted to Dr. J. Paget Stanfield, paediatrician at the M.R.C. unit. The study required co-operation between physician and psychologist, and I have been very lucky to work with such a kind and sincere person and have benefited greatly from his experience. Any credit for the investigation should go equally to him.

I am also grateful to our assistants, Mr. Y. Semindi and Mr. L. Mukasa, who despite illness and times of upheaval always succeeded in finding more former patients. Mrs. J. Kabanda and Mrs. I. Kasirye were competent interpreters, and were very kind and patient with the children and their parents; they guided me carefully as to the correct behaviour in rural Buganda.

The following persons also contributed to the study: Ms. I. Rutishauser, senior nutritionist at the M.R.C. unit, took the anthropometric measurements; Prof. and Dr. Herb and Anne Pick, Dr. Michael Okonji, and Dr. Neil Warren, all formerly of the Department of Social Psychology at Makerere University, extensively discussed and advised on the design of the study.

Finally, I wish to express my thanks to the staff members of the African Studies Centre and the University of Leiden who have, in many ways, helped me with the preparation of this monograph.

Contents

List of Tables, Appendices and Figures

Tables

Appendices

Figures

Introduction

Anyone who has ever seen a severely malnourished child cannot but wonder how this experience will have affected the child for the rest of its life. The misery and bodily disfigurements from which these children suffer leave the strong impression that they will never be quite normal again; that they will never be able to fulfil their human potential. In the last decade, attention has more and more become focused on the implications of malnutrition for brain growth and for the development of intellectual abilities. Sometimes extravagant claims have been made about the damage suffered by these children, but these claims were often based upon the results of studies with animals, in particular rats. Unreserved extrapolation of such findings to man is apt to be misleading because the development of the brain in relation to birth is very different in man. Also, the conditions to which these animals were often exposed generally fall outside the human experience.

This monograph is concerned with the relation between protein-energy malnutrition and intellectual abilities in man. Research into this question is bedevilled by problems of design and problems of measurement, both of nutritional status and of intellectual abilities. For this reason there is some pessimism about the feasibility and usefulness of, at least, small-scale studies and a tendency rather to concentrate on large, longitudinal investigations. We do not share this view because such undertakings have other, comparable weaknesses.

Although the reviews of this field of research by now probably surpass the actual number of empirical studies, a coherent framework accommodating most of the psychological evidence is still lacking. In this monograph such a framework is developed against a background of the results obtained in a study carried out jointly by Dr. J. Paget Stanfield, a paediatrician, and the author, who is a psychologist.

These findings concern a group of 60 Ugandan boys and girls who became severely malnourished during the first 27 months of life, resulting in their admission to the hospital. At the time of the study, the children varied in age from 11 to 17 years. The relation between malnutrition and intellectual abilities is explored in two ways: first by comparison with a matched group of children who were not severely malnourished during the first years of life, and secondly by relating present intellectual abilities to the condition of each child on admission to the hospital. These findings shed light on the role of the different components and the timing of malnutrition and are discussed against the evidence from other psychological studies.

The plan of the monograph is as follows. The first chapter starts with a brief description of Uganda and its population and continues with a discussion of food and nutrition in the country, in particular the incidence and aetiology of protein-energy malnutrition in young children. Chapter 2 formulates some research questions that can be asked and elaborates upon the impediments that face investigations. The next chapter discusses some aspects of psychological testing in Africa, south of the Sahara, paying particular attention to studies pertaining to the structure of abilities of African children. The design and organization of our investigation are described in chapter 4, which also includes an analysis of the medical condition of the children on admission. The tests that were used, their construction or adaptation, and data concerning the reliability and validity of the tests are presented in chapter 5. The findings of our study and other studies regarding intellectual abilities in the aftermath of malnutrition are discussed in chapter 6, together with the role of the components and the timing of malnutrition. Chapter 7 presents analogous findings concerning the motor ability of the Ugandan children, while in chapter 8 some aspects of the daily behaviour of these children are discussed. The argument that is developed in these chapters is compared with other recent findings and with some alternative explanations in chapter 9. This final chapter concludes with some speculations concerning the avenues by which malnutrition precisely interferes with intellectual abilities and with a brief discussion of the case for intervention.

Woubrugge,
November 1975

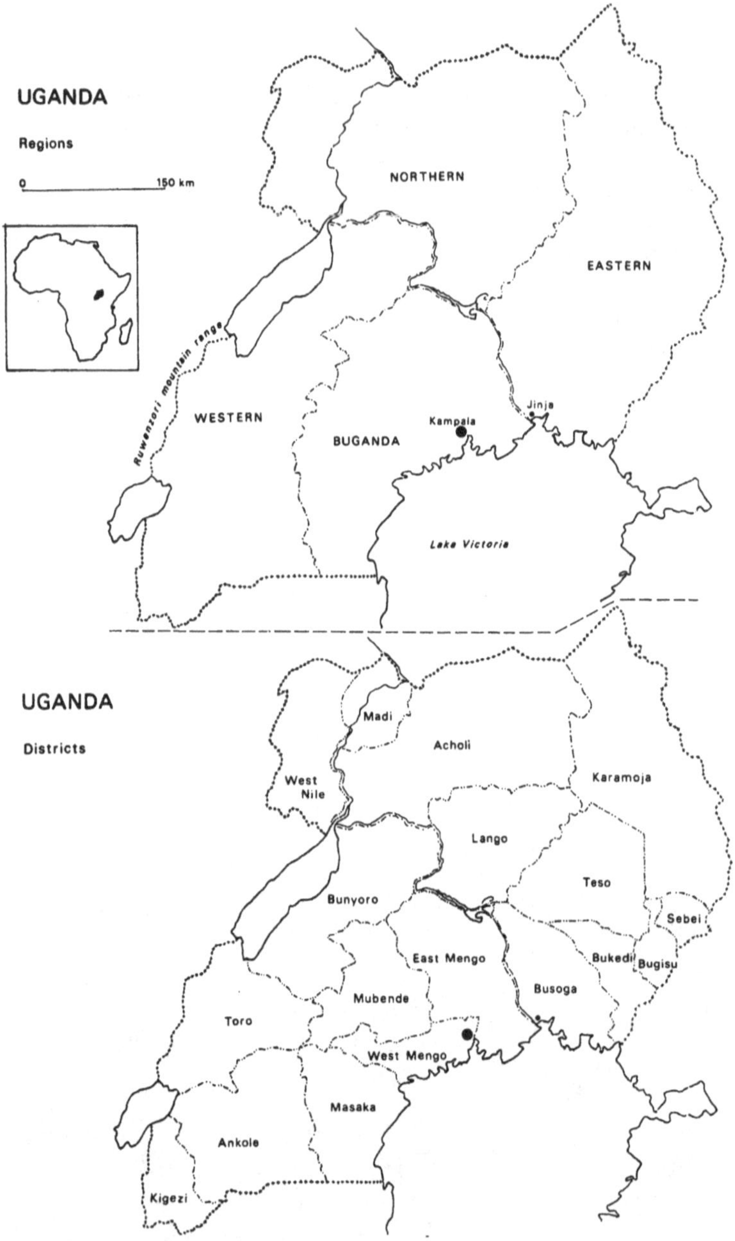

Figure 1 Uganda: regions and districts

1. Protein-Energy Malnutrition in Uganda

Uganda lies in the centre of Africa, north and northwest of Lake Victoria, the largest inland lake of Africa. Most of the country forms part of a high plateau. The altitude ranges from 750 to 1100 m in the northern plains, rising to 1400 m in the hilly country near Lake Victoria and further towards the south to hills of even 1800 or 2000 m in Ankole and Kigezi. The East African rift runs through the west of the country passing by the Ruwenzori mountain range.

The country is well endowed in respect of climate and soil. Although it lies on the equator, the high altitude and the presence of the vast water mass of Lake Victoria make for a rather moderate climate in the south. The north is, however, hotter than the rest of the country. Rainfall averages around 1250 mm per year throughout most of the country, with the exception of Karamoja district which is a much drier area. The country is characterized by wooded savannahs and grasslands, and the soils, in general, are fertile under the prevailing conditions.

Because of the distance to the sea and the relative inaccessibility of the territory, the first visitors from outside the continent reached the country only around the middle of the nineteenth century. Arab traders (and slavers) were soon followed by European explorers and missionaries. No sooner did Islam, Protestantism, and Catholicism gain footholds in the country than the missionaries became involved in internecine strife. At that time there was, of course, no country named Uganda; but a large number of tribes lived in the territory, each with its own political organization. There were large kingdoms such as Buganda and Kitara and smaller princedoms such as Ankole and Busoga. In other tribes, mainly those in the north, lineage groups and age sets formed the most important element of the political organization. The territory was proclaimed a British protectorate in 1894 but, contrary to what happened in neighbouring Kenya, Europeans were discouraged from settling in Uganda by the protectorate governments. Each of the tribes reacted in its own way to the imposition of central rule. The centre of trade and, later of government, soon lay with the largest and most powerful tribe, the Baganda, who live in the centre of the country in Buganda. Later, the capital, Kampala, also came to be situated here.

At the time of independence, in 1962, a semi-federal form of government was introduced in an effort to assure a balance between the interests of the different tribes, particularly between the north and the south. Mutesa, the Kabaka or traditional ruler of the Baganda, became the first president of the country while the northerner, Obote, became prime minister. Conflicts reflecting the antagonism between the different groups represented by these men soon arose and finally erupted into armed conflict in 1966. The Kabaka fled from the country, and Obote ruled until he, in turn, was deposed by the army commander, Amin, in 1971.

1.1 Population[1]

At the time of the 1969 population census, the African population of Uganda was 9.5 million, and it is estimated that it will reach 12 million in 1976. The country is divided into four administrative regions which are again divided into 18 districts (see map on page XVIII). Bantu tribes comprise 60 to 70% of the African population and inhabit the Western, the Buganda, and the southern part of the Eastern region. The Northern region and the north of the Eastern region are inhabited by Nilo-Hamitic and Nilotic tribes, each of these two groups comprising about 15% of the African population. The large number of individual tribes is illustrated by the fact that in 1959 the Baganda numbered one million people, and the next four tribes (the Banyankore, the Basoga, the Bakiga, and the Iteso) each numbered about half a million. At that time, three more tribes had more than 300,000 members, ten other tribes more than 100,000 members and a further nine tribes more than 33,000 people. The population density varies from 67 per km^2 in the Eastern region and 65 per km^2 in the Buganda region to 54 per km^2 in the Western region. The Northern region is less densely populated, with 29 inhabitants per km^2. Within the regions, population density also varies considerably. Bugisu and Bukedi districts in the Eastern region have 171 and 116 people per km^2, while Karamoja district has only 10 people per km^2. Karamoja has a distinct physical habitat in Uganda: the district is dry with sparse vegetation and is largely inhabited by pastoralists. In the Western region, Bunyoro has a population density of 35 and Kigezi of 127 inhabitants per km^2.

The large majority of the population lives in rural areas and there are few sizeable towns. The capital, Kampala, has a population of 330,000 people but the second town of the country, Jinja, numbers only 52,000 inhabitants. Ten more towns number more than 10,000 people. In 1969 only 7% of the population lived in towns with more than 2000 inhabitants.

Of the African population 19.3% are 4 years of age or younger and 26.9% are between 5 and 14 years of age. This age distribution, so characteristic of African countries, not only means that a large part of the population is unproductive but also that the adult population, in particular the women, are heavily burdened with the care and upbringing of these children. The birth rate is 49 per 1000 inhabitants per year and by the time a woman reaches 45 years of age she has on average given birth to 7 children. Of these babies 12 out of every 100 die before they reach their first birthday. The birth rate and the infant death rate are highest in parts of the north and the west of the country. The natural population increase is estimated at 3% per year.

While the educational level of the population compares favourably with that of other African countries, 62% of the African population of over 4 years of age have never had any formal education, that is 51% of the men and 73% of the women. In Karamoja district, however, 95% of the population over 4 years of age have never attended school. The Buganda region compares favourably with the rest of the country, for here 'only' 46% of the population never attended primary education. For those who attended primary schools, education has generally been limited to only a few years. Since these figures include younger as well as older generations, present school attendance rates are higher. In 1970 school enrolment as a percentage of the total primary school age groups was 52% (Uganda Government, 1972).

1.2 Agriculture, food, and nutrition

Uganda has few mineral deposits and little industry so that it is dependent mainly upon the rural production sector, in particular upon agriculture. Agricultural products comprised 79% of exports in 1969. The subsistence production contributed 30% to the gross domestic product in 1969, and commercial agricultural production contributed a further 25%. More significant is the fact that 90% of the population are dependent on the rural production sector for their livelihood (Uganda Government, 1972). The major cash crops are coffee and cotton. Cotton is grown mainly in the east and the north, whereas coffee is grown to the south in the areas alongside Lake Victoria. Both cash crops are grown largely by individual farmers and their families on smallholdings where they also grow food crops for their own consumption (*Atlas of Uganda*, 1967).

The main food crop among the Bantu tribes in the south is bananas, with sweet potatoes and cassava serving as alternative staple foods. Among the Nilotic and Nilo-Hamitic people in the north, millet and cassava are the most popular foods. Millet is the staple food of the Nilo-Hamitic tribes, while cassava is consumed primarily by the Nilotic tribes. Here, sweet potatoes also serve to vary or supplement the staple diet. Legumes such as groundnuts, beans, and peas are grown in lesser quantities throughout the country but least in the northern region (*Atlas of Uganda*, 1967; McDowell, 1972).

Meals usually consist of a staple food (bananas, cassava, sweet potatoes, millet) as the central dish, together with a relish that may consist of legumes, vegetables, and occasionally animal products. The energy value (calories) and protein content of various foodstuffs per 100 g of edible portion are presented in table 1. As regards the staple foods, bananas and sweet potatoes are very low in both calorie and protein content. Cassava flour contains more calories but equally few proteins, and when eaten fresh, the calorie content is as low as that of sweet potatoes. Finger millet, the only cereal, is the most nutritious of the staple foods. The legumes provide far richer sources of nutrients in terms of both calories and proteins. Vegetables, in general, are low in calories as well as in proteins. Where bananas, sweet potatoes, or cassava form the main components of the diet, the individual must consume large amounts of food to meet his nutritional requirements. It is evident that the legume relishes form an important source, not only of proteins but also of calories.

Table 1 *Nutrient content of various foodstuffs (per 100 grams of edible portion)*

	Calories	Proteins (grams)
Staple foods:		
bananas, cooking	100	1.5
sweet potato	166	1.3
cassava flour	350	1.8
finger millet meal	346	8.7
Legumes:		
groundnuts, shelled	577	27.1
beans, dry, mixed	330	19.5
cow pea	330	22.4
Vegetables:		
cabbage	23	1.5
onion	48	1.5
tomatoes	20	1.0

Source: Burgess and Burgess (1972).

As we shall learn later, small children often consume little of these relishes.

For the country and the population as a whole, the food availability and food requirements seem fairly well-balanced. Cleave (1972) has calculated that on average, 2140 calories and 52.5 grams of proteins are required *per capita* per day. Previous estimates of the food that is available in Uganda have been rather high, ranging from 3700 calories (Gale, 1960) to 5200 calories (MacDonald, 1963) *per capita* per day, which raised the question whether the Ugandan farmers were overproducing or whether these were perhaps overestimates. Recent estimates, after the F.A.O. agricultural census in 1960, arrive at much lower figures. Cleave (1972) has calculated that in 1963, 2289 calories and 56.6 grams of proteins were available *per capita* per day, and this author also estimated that in periods of need, an additional 400 calories would be available, mainly from food that is otherwise not harvested. McDowell (1972) estimated that on the basis of the main food crops, excluding vegetables and animal products, 2825 calories and 55.9 grams of proteins were available *per capita* per day in 1968. These calculations suggest that the requirements and availability of food in terms of calories and proteins are reasonably matched. Uganda is generally not regarded as being threatened by food shortages (May and McLellan, 1970). F.A.O. does, however, recommend that the target for protein production in a country should lie 20% above what is required. According to Cleave (1972), in Uganda that target (which should be 63 grams of proteins *per capita* per day) is not reached.

Computations on a national basis do not reveal the possible maldistribution of food, such as may, for example, occur between geographical regions or between age groups. McDowell (1972) has estimated the food availability in the four regions on the basis of the main food crops (excluding Karamoja and Toro district for which no figures were available). The Buganda and Western regions come off poorest with, respectively, 1588 and 1973 calories and 33 and 46 grams of proteins available *per capita* per day. The population of the Eastern region appears to be much better off with 3548 calories and 66 grams of proteins *per capita* per day, while in the Northern region the figures are

4625 calories and 82 grams of proteins. It must be pointed out that the north and the east have seasonal harvests, and foods have to be stored. This storage leads to wastage and greater losses than in the Buganda and Western regions where a more continuous food supply is found. Nevertheless, the figures suggest a potential deficit in both calories and proteins in the Buganda and Western regions, where the balance between requirements and availability seems precarious.

Adult starvation, however, is rare in the country, with the exception of Karamoja district.[2] In the rest of the country, adult malnutrition occurs only incidentally, and when it does occur, it seems to result from a breakdown of the traditional forms of care for the old and the infirm rather than from an actual shortage of food (Bennett and Stanfield, 1971, p. 6). The vulnerable group of infants and young children, however, is in greater danger.

1.3 The incidence of protein-energy malnutrition of early childhood

Protein-energy malnutrition of early childhood ranges from mild and moderate forms, to the severe degrees of kwashiorkor, marasmus, and mixed syndromes. Kwashiorkor patients are generally characterized by oedema, muscle wasting, and severe apathy, while hair and skin changes also occur frequently. Marasmic patients are characterized primarily by extreme wasting: the child is mere skin and bones. Although far less active than healthy children, marasmic patients do not show such pronounced apathy as kwashiorkor patients. Generally, kwashiorkor is associated with a diet that is primarily deficient in proteins, whereas marasmus is attributed to a diet that is deficient principally in calories, but also in proteins. Most malnourished children in Uganda, however, present severe mixed syndromes or, more usually, mild to moderate forms which defy precise classification (Jelliffe and Stanfield, 1966). Throughout this book, malnutrition, childhood malnutrition and protein-energy malnutrition are used to refer to the general condition and include mild, moderate, and severe forms. In accord with recent usage the term protein-energy malnutrition is used instead of protein-calorie malnutrition.

Uganda, like many African countries, has to cope with a high incidence rate of malnutrition among its young children, as the results of various surveys show. Burgess (1962a, b, c, d, e) determined the total number of children under five years of age who suffered from kwashiorkor or marasmus and who were seen at dispensaries or admitted to hospitals in five districts during the course of one year. This number of children was expressed as a percentage of the total number of children between 8 months and five years of age who lived in each district (Dean and Burgess, 1962). These percentages[3] are as follows:

Busoga	1.3%
Bukedi	1.2%
Bugisu	0.9%
Kigezi	0.9%
Ankole	0.5%

These figures are, in all likelihood, underestimates of the actual incidence of malnutrition among young children. Those children who were malnourished but who never attended a dispensary were not counted. Furthermore, only children with severe malnutrition were recorded, but many more children show some signs of malnutrition.

In fact, previous surveys by Gongora and McFie (1959) reported much higher rates of incidence. In these surveys was recorded the number of children under six years of age who suffered from kwashiorkor or marasmus and who were seen at selected dispensaries in various districts over a period of, on average, eight weeks. In this case, this total was expressed as a percentage of the number of children who attended the dispensaries during the same period. These percentages for the districts were the following:

Busoga	7.0%	Kigezi	6.4%	Mubende	17.6%
Bukedi	14.5%	Mengo	11.2%	Bunyoro	8.7%
Bugisu	5.6%	Masaka	5.4%	Toro	4.7%

The previous investigations did not cover the northern districts of the country. Jelliffe and others carried out surveys in selected villages in West Nile (1962), Acholi (1963), and Karamoja (1964) districts. In West Nile all children under four years, in Acholi all children under five years, and in Karamoja all 'pre-school' children living in the villages were examined. The incidence of severe malnutrition among these children was 1.0-1.1% in all three areas. The incidence of children with low weights was much higher. In West Nile and Acholi, 6.6% and 4.3% of the children fell below 60% of the mean weights of healthy Baganda children which, according to the Gomez classification, qualifies them as suffering from third degree malnutrition. Many more children, 75% and 63% respectively, weighed less than 90% of this local standard (first degree malnutrition according to the Gomez classification). It must be pointed out that the Baganda standards are not necessarily applicable to these groups, so that some caution must be exercised in the interpretation of these figures. A similar survey was carried out in Kigezi district (Jelliffe *et al.*, 1961) and here 1.5% of the children under four years suffered from severe malnutrition, while 43% fell below 90% of the Baganda standard.

The fact that the percentages of severe malnutrition reported by Jelliffe and his co-workers in these surveys hover around 1%, just as in Burgess's (1962a, b, c, d, e) surveys, is misleading because the first were point-prevalence surveys (recording the number of children who suffered from severe malnutrition at one particular point in time), whereas Burgess's records cover one full year. Jelliffe's findings, therefore, point to a higher incidence of severe malnutrition than the figures presented by Burgess. As has already been mentioned, the latter findings are probably underestimates. Rutishauser (1971) comments that although Gongora and McFie (1959) must have labelled relatively mild cases as severe malnutrition to arrive at their much higher estimates, these figures may nevertheless reflect the much higher rate of incidence of children with some signs of malnutrition. There are in fact indications that this incidence rate may even be higher. The findings by Jelliffe indicate that at any one time, 40% or more of the children suffered from first degree of malnutrition, since their weights fell below 90% of the local weight standard. The results of two biochemical tests among selected groups of children under 4 years of age in Buganda and Bukedi showed signs of malnutrition in 32-47% of the cases, although the incidence of severe malnutrition was less than 1% in both groups (Rutishauser and Whitehead, 1969). This evidence suggests that it may well be 'that nearly every child in Uganda goes through a phase of marginal malnutrition or delayed growth at some time during the first four years of life.' (Rutishauser, 1971, p. 15.) A conservative estimate would be that at least 1% of the children under 5 years of age suffer from severe malnutrition each year, which in 1969 would have meant 18,000 children. Contrary to what might have been expected from the previous data on food availability, it appears that childhood malnutrition occurs all over the country and is not limited to particular geographical regions.

1.4 The aetiology of childhood malnutrition

The reasons for the prevalence of malnutrition among young children in Uganda are complex. The immediate causative factors are well known: dietary inadequacy and infections. In recent years the important role that infections play has been increasingly realized. Brown and Opio (1966), for example, found that 40% of the children admitted with kwashiorkor to Mulago Hospital in Kampala during one year also suffered from infections. Infections not only contribute to growth faltering and loss of weight but also negatively interfere with certain metabolic processes (Frood, Whitehead, and Coward, 1971). The incidence of infections among young children in Africa generally needs no further illustration; it results from, among other things, poor sanitary conditions and the lack of clean water (Bennett and Stanfield, 1971).

The young child has a limited capacity to consume food and is in need of a diet which is relatively high in calories. At the same time the child needs relatively more proteins than the adult to sustain growth. Provided that the mother has sufficient breast milk, the child usually fares well till the age of six months. After that age, breast milk alone is insufficient to meet the nutritional needs of the child. In many African societies supplementary feeding is traditionally introduced about this age and usually consists of portions of the adult diet. About the age of one year, or earlier if the mother becomes pregnant again, the child is weaned. The task then confronting the child is clearly illustrated in the following passage:

> The normal meal pattern is usually of a central dish of the staple which is eaten with savoury sauces made from legumes, green vegetables and, occasionally, meat or fish. ... Tough 'chewy' meat is favoured and fish is normally cooked whole with the bones. These practices restrict the availability of these foods to young children who cannot easily masticate the meat and who will not be given fish because of the presence of bones. In these circumstances the young children may receive only the liquid in which the meat, fish or legumes have been cooked. Some legumes, particularly beans, which are often cooked in their stews are indigestible so far as young children are concerned and may cause diarrhoea.
>
> Children are also expected to fend for themselves at a fairly early age. Immediately after weaning the child may be set down at the adult meal and, although, at the outset, may be fed with portions of the staple dipped into the sauce by the mother or older children, he will be expected to eat by himself very quickly. In these circumstances the child's diet is likely to consist mainly of the staple and as much of the sauce as he can manage to mop up. ...
>
> In general the only concession towards special requirements for children's foods relates to texture since it is recognised that young children should have soft or smooth foods. All too often this can result in extensive use of starchy low-protein foods such as bananas, cassava or sweet potatoes and, in these cases, the bulky nature of the food can result in repletion of appetite before nutritional requirements are met. (McDowell, 1972, pp. 149-50.)

The dangers of such a low calorie/low protein diet are enhanced by the usual pattern of meals in most homes. The Padhola household described below may serve as an example of many other households in the country.

> Meal patterns vary at different times of the year, since they are closely related to patterns of work. There is a tendency to have the same number of meals each day, namely a snack early in the morning and two main meals during the day, but the timing changes. Cultivating is started early in the morning. Before the adults leave the house they may drink tea or eat some of the cold food from the evening meal, but often they start without 'breakfast'. Cold food is thought to be bad for children, to upset their stomaches and make them ill, but nevertheless, it is they who usually eat the left over food. After returning from the fields, the wife prepares the first main meal of the day. A main meal should consist of a staple and a relish, but sometimes only a staple is eaten with salt and water. When farm work continues late into the day, this may be the only meal that is eaten if preparation takes a long time. In this case, a snack may be eaten on returning from the fields, while waiting for the meal. Alternatively the first meal may consist of some dish which is quick to prepare. When a second meal is prepared in the evening, after a late first meal, the younger children are often asleep before it is ready. (Sharman, 1972, p. 81.)

Dietary inadequacy and infections are the general reasons for the relatively low nutritional status of many Ugandan children. A vicious circle, in which poor nutrition leads to a decreased resistance against infections which in turn lead to a poor nutritional status, lays the basis for acute malnutrition.

The puzzling fact remains that, under these circumstances, some children develop severe malnutrition, some show only some signs of malnutrition, while others even appear to thrive. This has made researchers look for other contributing factors that negatively influence the diet. Obviously, extreme conditions such as child neglect and exceptional poverty will have a bearing on the diet and the condition of children. However, it remains to be seen how much of the variation in the nutritional status of Ugandan children can be attributed to variations in conditions other than the incidence and frequency of infections. The two factors that are most often mentioned are first, poverty, and second, instability of the relation between mother and child and instability of the family.

The role of poverty in the causation of malnutrition in Uganda is often considered as self-evident but there are, in fact, few data to support this view. Welbourn (1955), in a study of 65 kwashiorkor patients, reported that none of the families of these children appeared poorer than its neighbours, while many of the families were comparatively well-to-do. In another study, the poverty of the family was considered an important cause in only 4 out of 28 kwashiorkor patients (Farmer, 1960). The relation between the socio-economic level and childhood malnutrition was studied in detail among the Padhola in Bukedi district. Families that were well-to-do, according to their cash income, were found to have a greater consumption of high-protein relishes, a lower consumption of green vegetables, and fewer occasions on which no relish was served at all (Sharman, 1972, p. 83). Despite this positive relation between socio-economic level and protein consumption by the family, there was no relation between it and the nutritional status of the children. Malnourished children were just as frequent among the well-to-do families as they were among the poorer families. This lack of evidence for a relation between socio-economic level and childhood malnutrition is not surprising when it is realized that in a subsistence economy, nearly every family grows its own food and that poverty eludes definition. It may be argued that poverty among immigrant groups, such as the Rwanda and the Luo, is very different because these groups have less access to land. Their position is such that they are less able or unable to grow their own foods, and since they are dependent on the cash economy they are, in fact, much poorer than people who manage to grow their own foodcrops. Indeed, some studies point to a somewhat higher incidence of malnutrition among the Rwanda but not among the Luo (Brown and Opio, 1966; Welbourn, 1959).

Other factors that are often held responsible for childhood malnutrition are instability of the relation between mother and child and instability of the family. A disturbance of the mother-child relation is also suggested by some of the local descriptions of the disease. The common Luganda word for malnutrition, 'obwosi', implies that it occurs in the child when the mother becomes pregnant again. The 'heat' of the unborn child in the mother's womb is considered to be a danger to the lastborn child. This child is therefore weaned and may even be sent away to live with relatives. The Padhola recognize a similar cause for malnutrition. 'Ther', as they call it, occurs when the mother becomes pregnant again, while the child is still on the breast and consequently has to be weaned (Sharman, 1972, p. 78). Of course, the very word 'kwashiorkor' derives from the language of the Ga in Ghana and refers to the illness that the elder child gets when the next child is born (Williams, 1935). Two aspects, in particular, have drawn the attention of various authors: that of 'sudden' weaning and that of sending the child to live with relatives.

'Sudden' weaning, the sudden and complete denial of the breast, on a day fixed in advance, is supposedly widely practised throughout Uganda, but particularly among the Baganda upon whom most authors base their observations. This kind of weaning is regarded as a serious shock for the child who recovers from it only with the greatest difficulty (Welbourn, 1955, p. 102). The term, 'sudden' weaning, suggests an abrupt transition from a breast milk diet to solid foods. According to Ainsworth (1967) in her detailed study of infancy in Buganda, such weaning is the exception rather than the rule. Traditionally, and today, additional foods are introduced when the child is still on the breast, usually around the age of six months. In the old days the actual weaning at 2 or 3 years of age is reported to have been abrupt in that the breast which had previously been available on demand, was suddenly and completely denied to the child (Ainsworth, 1967, p. 403). But nowadays, weaning occurs around one year of age and is usually gradual in that breastfeeding is at first reduced during the day, but at night the child is still given access to the breast (Ainsworth, 1967, p. 406). There is, however, a group of children who for various reasons (e.g. lactation failure, pregnancy of the mother, or death of the mother) are weaned early and suddenly. There are some indications that these children are vulnerable. Among a group of 51 kwashiorkor patients whose lactational history was recorded, 13 (25%) had been weaned before 12 months of age because of their mothers' pregnancies. Among a comparison group consisting of 326 children that were not malnourished, only 22 (7%) shared such an experience (Welbourn, 1959). It seems likely that in these cases the early weaning poses the greatest danger.

The sending of children to relatives has created considerable confusion among researchers since two practices have often been mistaken (Ainsworth, 1967, p. 418). There was, among the Baganda, a practice of sending the child away to the grandmother at weaning, but the child was returned to the mother after one or two nights to assure its well-being. The other practice is to send the child away later on to live with relatives for various (not necessarily negative) reasons. How does this practice relate to the occurrence of malnutrition in children?

Investigations reveal that between 7% and 22% of kwashiorkor patients who were seen at a hospital, a dispensary, and a nutrition unit, were living away from their parents (Brown and Opio, 1966; Farmer, 1960; Schneideman, Bennett and Rutishauser, 1971). The incidence of this practice among the general child population was, however, assessed in only one investigation. Welbourn (1959) found that 12 (18%) out of 65 kwashiorkor patients who were seen at various child welfare clinics near Kampala were living away from home, but that this practice was limited largely to the Baganda children. Among the 24 Baganda kwashiorkor patients, 11 (46%) were living away from home, while this was the case for only 23 (9%) of 248 Baganda children who also attended these clinics but who were not malnourished. A straightforward conclusion is difficult to draw since only one of the malnourished children lived in town whereas 82 (33%) of the 248 comparison children lived there. One study indicates that in one rural area 26% of the children under the age of 5 were living with relatives (Welbourn, 1963). Nevertheless, these results suggest that this practice contributes to the occurrence of malnutrition in young children, at least among the Baganda. From these figures, it does not become clear whether the children were being sent away voluntarily or whether the separation coincided with a separation between the parents.

In fact, family instability is often mentioned as a contributing factor on its own. Where father and mother are separated or where a child is born out of wedlock, a cohesive family is presumedly lacking, which will have negative consequences for the child. Such superficial observations overlook the intricate network of family relations and obligations upon which an individual in an African society can often fall back. It also overlooks that where marriages are frequently broken, they are also frequently engaged in. Two investigations (Farmer, 1960; Brown and Opio, 1966) reported an incidence of at least 14-19% of broken marriages among the parents of kwashiorkor patients. Welbourn (1959) found that the parents of 9 (14%) out of 65 kwashiorkor patients had separated, but that this was the case among only 35 (7%) out of 507 well-nourished children. Schneideman and others (1971), reported an even higher incidence (37%) of broken families among the children who attended a nutrition rehabilitation unit in Kampala. It is not clear whether the last authors used the same definition of a broken family as the previous authors, while comparison data for non-malnourished children are, unfortunately, lacking.

1.5 Conclusion

Although enough food is grown in Uganda to provide for the population, many children suffer from different degrees of protein-energy malnutrition. Each year, at least 1% of the children under 5 years of age may suffer from severe malnutrition, which in 1969 alone meant 18,000 children. In addition, many more children show growth retardation or other signs of malnutrition, and it is likely that nearly every child goes through such a phase during the first four years of life. Among children with severe malnutrition who were admitted to hospitals in Uganda, a mortality rate of around 20% has been observed (Wharton, 1971). The mortality rate of untreated severe malnutrition is unknown but may be as high as 50% (Sai, 1972, p. 141; Bengoa, 1973). The number of children who died from malnutrition in Uganda between 1960 and 1963 has been estimated at between 5000 and 7000 each year (Wharton, 1971). Malnutrition is also a contributing factor in the severity and consequent mortality rates of other diseases.

Childhood malnutrition in Uganda springs from the vicious circle of frequent infections and inadequate diet which nearly every child experiences. This in itself may be enough to cause growth retardation and even severe malnutrition in otherwise normal children, living in ordinary circumstances. In a number of cases, however, other factors, such as early weaning, marital instability, the incidental practice among the Baganda of sending the child away from home, and poverty among immigrant groups, may aggravate the condition of the child.

For both the child and its mother, an episode of severe malnutrition means a period of intense suffering. The child is listless or apathetic (Geber and Dean, 1956), usually immersed in its misery, while the mother is often at her wit's end, powerless to help the child. The moderate and mild forms of malnutrition also influence a child's vitality and his behaviour (Rutishauser and Whitehead, 1972), while great efforts and extreme care are required from the mother to help the child through its frequent illnesses from which he or she never seems to recover quite fully.

What about the children who live through an episode of severe malnutrition? It seems fairly well established that they suffer a permanent growth retardation, but whether this in itself is a bad thing is not clear. There are also indications that certain organs, such as the liver and the pancreas, are affected, although the permanency of the damage is uncertain, as is the effect on the child's general health and his chances for life (Stanfield, 1972). The most serious consequences ascribed to malnutrition are that brain growth is affected and that this leads to a lowered intellectual capacity in these children. These are really two different statements that should be properly distinguished: the first, that malnutrition damages the brain; the second, that malnutrition results in lowered intellectual abilities. This monograph concentrates on the relation between protein-energy malnutrition in early childhood and intellectual abilities later in life. Before the particulars of our study are presented, the problems inherent to this field of research and the experience that has been gained with the testing of intellectual abilities in Africa are discussed in the next two chapters.

2. Impediments in Design and Method

There is increasing evidence, on the basis of animal and human studies, that protein-energy malnutrition in early childhood impairs mental development. We shall not review the evidence from animal studies, but it has long been known that malnutrition impairs the somatic growth of many species. It has also been shown that certain types of malnutrition, induced during the period of most rapid brain growth in animals, interfere with the development of the central nervous system and may result in smaller brains, lower brain weights, and reductions in DNA content, cell number, and cell size (see Cheek, Holt and Mellits, 1972; Birch, 1972; and Frankova, 1974, for reviews). The behavioural implications of early growth restrictions in animals are discussed by Dobbing and Smart (1974).

At first sight, the evidence from studies with children seems hardly less convincing. Autopsies on Ugandan children who had died from malnutrition before the age of 4 years revealed reductions in brain weight of 10-15% (Brown, 1966). The brains of children who had died of marasmus during the first years of life showed large reductions in cell number, varying from 15% to 60% (Winick, Brasel, and Rosso, 1972, p. 31). Many psychological studies of the survivors of acute malnutrition report that, later in life, these children fall behind their peers in test performance. For various reasons, reviewers are very hesitant to draw definite conclusions. Frisch speaks of 'surmises' that 'should not be treated as facts' (1970, p. 194) and Warren regards the 'influence of malnutrition on mental development ... a rather open question.' (1973, p. 324.) Some are convinced of the deleterious influence of malnutrition on mental development (Birch, 1972, p. 781); but others point to the need for unravelling the various factors influencing a child's development, rather than taking malnutrition as the single focus of research (Klein, Habicht, and Yarbrough, 1971, p. 87). After a recent symposium on 'Early malnutrition and mental development' it was concluded that 'despite of the widely held and widely publicized opinion that malnutrition in early life jeopardizes mental development the evidence to support this opinion – especially from studies conducted in man – is scanty' (W.H.O., 1974, p. 101). This hesitation finds its cause in some (apparently) conflicting findings, but results mainly from the imperfections and inevitable limitations of the studies in this field, limitations that will be discussed in this chapter. First it must be pointed out that the question whether 'malnutrition influences mental development' is too general to lend itself to fruitful investigation and requires further qualifications.

2.1 The research questions

Protein-energy malnutrition (P.E.M.) of early childhood is a complex of elements, the most important of which include severity (whether subclinical or overt), duration (whether acute, chronic, or relapsing), and metabolic disturbance (whether oedematous (hypoproteinaemic) or marasmic). Children also suffer from malnutrition at different ages, and the illness often coincides with infections or other deficiencies. Many of these elements are interrelated. In the typical case, malnutrition starts during the first year of life with growth faltering, caused by an insufficiency of calories and proteins, associated with frequent infections. As this process continues the child becomes increasingly 'marasmic'. At any time a variety of acute stresses, including infections and further reductions in the intake of proteins and calories, may precipitate an acute metabolic imbalance of the child and result in 'kwashiorkor'. One can therefore distinguish in any severely malnourished child a varying mixture of chronic undernutrition and acute malnutrition. The first is reflected mainly in the stunting of somatic growth; the second, in metabolic abnormalities, chief of which are hypoproteinaemia and oedema. It is conceivable that only certain patterns of protein-energy malnutrition will influence mental development or that they have different effects. It has been suggested that marasmus is more damaging than kwashiorkor, but it is unclear whether the chronic nature of the illness or the younger age group in which it usually occurs should be held responsible for this (Scrimshaw and Gordon, 1968, p. 289). Similarly, it has been suggested, by analogy with the results of animal studies, that the more malnutrition coincides with the period of fastest brain growth during the first few months of life, the greater the damage may turn out to be (Dobbing, 1968, p. 196). Recent insights put more emphasis on the different stages of the brain-growth spurt (Dobbing, 1974). It is equally possible that chronic, subclinical malnutrition is more damaging than a brief, acute attack by itself – or vice versa. Thus there is a need for specific hypotheses regarding the nature of the illness and its possible effects, whereas many studies until now have been limited to a general syndrome of malnutrition.

The mode of influence by which malnutrition affects mental development also merits attention. Different processes, which may operate simultaneously, have been postulated. Malnutrition may distort brain structure during growth: the 'brain damage' hypothesis. Malnutrition also results in apathy and the consequent lack of experience and stimulation for the child, which may also result in intellectual impairment: the 'deprivation' hypothesis. Deprivation, however, may also affect brain structure, as Levitsky and Barnes (1975) have demonstrated with rats, where experiential deprivation resulted in histological and chemical changes in the brain. It has also been postulated that the motivation and the ability to concentrate of malnourished children may be primarily affected (Klein, Gilbert, Canosa, and De Leon, 1969).

The nature of the impairment also demands consideration. Is there a depression of intellectual functioning comparable to that of the generally retarded child; or are specific areas of cognitive functioning affected, such as verbal and language abilities; spatial-perceptual abilities; intersensory integration; or the abilities of memory, learning, and attention?

Furthermore, there is the question of the permanency of the effects. Most studies until now have been carried out within a few years of the episode of malnutrition, usually with children not much older than 7 years of age. Any retardation or deficit at this age may still be erased during the remainder of the children's growth and development, so that they may ultimately suffer no permanent consequences.

Many factors other than nutrition determine the course of a child's intellectual development. Some of these may accompany malnutrition, which raises the question of control.

2.2 Control

The fundamental restriction of all nutrition research with humans is that malnutrition can be only a naturally occurring phenomenon and may never be wilfully induced for research purposes. This excludes the possibility of controlled experiments. Research is limited to field studies in which malnutrition is observed in its natural surroundings, accompanied by other social and economic, possibly confounding, variables. Although true experiments are not possible, there exists a large variety of other designs that can be used. A primary requirement of most designs is to have a control or comparison group. A comparison group is necessary so that the effects on subjects of a certain event, such as an episode of malnutrition or nutrition intervention, can be compared with the changes occurring among subjects who have not experienced this event. In general, when such a comparison group is not included, differences (or lack of differences) between 'before' and 'after' conditions may result from other events occurring between the two measurements: from the maturation of subjects over time, or from increased familiarity with the taking of tests. In this particular field of investigation, however, comparison groups are especially required because a comparison of 'before' and 'after' conditions is factually impossible to carry out. Usually, malnutrition occurs between 6 months and 3 years of age, and since there are no good measures in existence for infants younger than 6 months which adequately predict their later intellectual abilities (Dureman, 1974; Tizard, 1974a), it is not possible to compare the intellectual abilities of these children with their abilities some years later. Therefore any effects must be observed in differences from adequate comparison groups. The selection of a meaningful comparison group is fraught with difficulties.

Investigators have repeatedly pointed out that malnutrition occurs typically in an environment of poverty and ignorance. Such an environment will in itself be detrimental to the optimal development of children, and any retardation may be attributed to other aspects of the environment as much as to the associated malnutrition. This association between malnutrition and a backward social environment seems particularly characteristic of the American continent, where malnutrition is largely a product of urban slum conditions and extreme rural poverty. In large parts of Africa, however, the distribution of malnutrition among the population is less closely connected with poverty but has an ecology of its own, as described for Uganda in the previous chapter. Nevertheless, any investigation into the relation between malnutrition and intellectual abilities must allow for a possible association between malnutrition and a poor social environment, both of which may negatively influence intellectual abilities. Consequently, research has continuously concentrated on trying to separate the effects of these two major hazards to the child's intellectual development.

Some studies have tried to achieve this by limiting the investigation to one, usually the poorer, segment of the population (Mönckeberg, Tisler, Toro, Gattas, and Vega, 1972). The implicit assumption is that within this group, socio-cultural differences are not large enough to result in variations in mental ability. Pollitt (1972), however, has reported that among such a group of Peruvian children test performance nevertheless correlated with other biological and social variables besides malnutrition. Often the investigators have resorted to matching procedures, whereby groups of previously malnourished children are compared with children who have not been malnourished, but who have the same social, economic, and educational background. The use of siblings who have not suffered from malnutrition is often recommended (Tizard, 1974b, p. 67) but merits special comment. Since siblings have been brought up in the same environment they have been exposed to the same influences. However, they may and will differ in sex, age, and education, and the premise that they have an identical home environment is also open to criticism. Birth rank and sex influence the position of the child at home, while the episode of malnutrition which one child suffered may have had a lasting influence on the rest of the family. More important is the fact that siblings may not be as different in nutritional history as is often assumed. Although they may not have suffered an episode of malnutrition requiring hospitalization, their general nutritional status may be similar, precisely because they have been raised in the same environment.

The necessity of manipulation of environmental variables, as in matching or analysis of covariance, depends very much upon which of the research questions formulated above is subject to investigation. An obvious way of achieving control over environmental variables lies in comparing different groups of malnourished children, e.g. children who have suffered at different ages or who have suffered from different types of malnutrition. This has two advantages. Since all the children have been malnourished, it is far less likely that they differ in their social background than when comparison children are used who have not been malnourished. Secondly, the research questions formulated will necessarily be more specific.

Where a study concentrates on the nature of an eventual impairment, an alternative method of comparison is to use developmental controls (Warren, 1970). The comparison of previously malnourished children with younger children of the same mental age shows whether malnourished children, although retarded, are cognitively similar to the normal child or whether they suffer specific deficits. The danger of this procedure lies in regression to the mean when repeated measurements are made over time (Campbell and Stanley, 1966). Furthermore, developmental controls must also be drawn from a similar social background lest specific deficits resulting from other causes are confounded with those resulting from malnutrition.

Warren (1970) has suggested the use of other comparison

groups, notably children who have suffered experiential deprivation through causes other than malnutriton, e.g. children in orphanages or bedridden patients. Such a comparison may shed light on the question of whether the deficits in malnourished children arise through deprivation or through distortion of brain growth; similarly, we may add, might comparison with children who are known to have suffered brain damage.

Finally, where the interest is only in the permanency of any effects, or a possible 'catch-up' occurring later in life, the developmental curves of malnourished children can be compared with those of any group of non-malnourished children because, in this case, one is interested in the growth curves, not in their absolute level. With the last possibility, however, one should bear in mind that theoretically a relation between the developmental curve and its absolute level cannot be ruled out.

2.3 Research designs

The numerous titles given to research designs in this particular field of investigation hold different meanings for different authors. The terms retrospective, prospective, longitudinal, semilongitudinal, cross-sectional, follow-up, ecological, intervention study, and various combinations of these are freely and confusingly used. This confusion is partly the result of the difference in nomenclature used in the medical and in the social sciences. To our knowledge, the distinction between prospective and retrospective studies is the following. In a retrospective study the starting point is the observation of an effect, and inquiries are then made about the suspected causes in the past. When, on the other hand, a particular illness is observed at the time that it occurs and its consequences are studied, the study is called prospective (Doll, 1959, p. 65; Barker and Bennett, 1973, p. 33). This qualifies virtually all the studies in this field as prospective, with one exception which we will describe below. The distinction between cross-sectional and longitudinal studies derives originally from descriptive studies of human growth.[4] Cross-sectional studies usually consist of extensive surveys of large samples of children which are examined only once. In longitudinal studies, a single group of children is repeatedly examined throughout the study. When applied not to descriptive growth studies but to studies of cause and effect, this distinction becomes less helpful. As soon as children are examined more than once, for example at the time of illness and again some years later, a study qualifies as longitudinal (Billewicz, 1974a, p. 53). This implies that virtually all studies in this field are longitudinal since most of them meet this requirement. In follow-up studies the researcher tries to find out what has happened to a group of patients after their discharge (Truelove, 1959, p. 92). The four basic designs that we will distinguish will be referred to as retrospective, follow-up, longitudinal, and intervention studies. It does not need to be emphasized that the meaning of these terms, as defined below, does not necessarily correspond to their use by other authors. These four designs do not exhaust all the studies that are possible or that have been carried out. Mixed forms are possible, but these four designs present the important characteristics of studies in this particular field of investigation.

2.4 Retrospective studies

The weakest design in terms of the conclusions that can be drawn is that of retrospective studies. In these studies, made later in the child's life, no observations have been made during early childhood. Previous malnutrition is inferred either from recollections by the parents or from a known outcome of malnutrition, such as stunting of somatic growth. Usually height is treated as the independent variable, under the assumption that differences in height reflect differences in nutritional history. Once height is found to be related to intellectual abilities, this leads to the inference that malnutrition affects mental development. Serious problems of interpretation face these studies. First, it is more than likely that height is influenced also by other biological and genetic factors, even in countries where malnutrition is endemic. Furthermore, even if the stunting of height reflects previous malnutrition, little or nothing is known about the nature, the duration, the severity, and the age of onset of the malnutrition. Lastly, this design leaves the serious possibility of confounding, environmental variables.

Cravioto, DeLicardie, and Birch (1966), in the well known study from Guatemala, tried to avoid this last problem by studying children from an upper-class, urban area and children from a poor, rural area. The authors argued that among the poor group stature differences would be determined predominantly by nutritional history, whereas other factors would operate in the upper-class group. Thus they expected differences between short and tall children on a sensory integration task in the rural group but not in the urban group. They conclude from their findings that this is indeed the case, and have subsequently been widely quoted. Closer inspection of their data, however, shows that in *both* the poor and the upper-class group the shorter children make many more errors than the taller children.[5]

Edwards and Craddock (1973) resorted to matching. They studied two groups of Australian aboriginal children who differed in head circumference, height, and weight but who had been individually matched on sex, age, and type of residence. These children were between 7 and 13 years of age. No information is presented regarding their formal education. The small children scored significantly below the big children on the L.M. Binet test. But even this study leaves the basic problems of this design unsolved: that is, do the height differences really reflect previous malnutrition and if so, what were the characteristics of the malnutrition?

2.5 Follow-up studies

To date, mainly follow-up and some longitudinal studies have been published. The individual studies and their findings will be described later on; here we will concern ourselves with a discussion of the strengths and weaknesses of these designs.

In follow-up studies children are usually selected on the basis of documented admission to hospitals or clinics for malnutrition. Thus antecedent nutritional data and observations exist. These children are traced (if necessary) and studied later in life.

One problem inherent to follow-up studies is the difficulty of finding a group of children which were not malnourished during childhood. To take a random group of children would be unacceptable because in countries where childhood malnutrition is endemic, it cannot be assumed that these children have not suffered from malnutrition in early childhood. It is necessary to have data on the nutritional status of all children in the study during that period.

The weaknesses of this design lie in the fact that for the malnourished children, there are usually no observations in existence prior to the admission and that there are also no observations for part or all of the years between the discharge and the study. Hence the possibility exists that both the previously malnourished and the comparison children may have suffered (again) during the intervening years from malnutrition, which had gone unnoticed. This possibility decreases after the age of 2.5 years because children are most vulnerable before that age. When matching is used in these studies, it is usually done with the help of the data collected at the time of the study, which does not necessarily guarantee that these data reflect the family situation at the time of malnutrition or during the intervening years. For this to result in systematic errors, it would require a systematic improvement in the socio-economic situation of the families of previously malnourished children *vis-à-vis* the families of children who have not suffered from malnutrition – and there is little reason to expect such a trend.

Before we move to the discussion of the longitudinal and intervention designs, the ethical implications of such investigations require consideration. In these studies children are usually observed before, during, and long after an episode of malnutrition. The question immediately arises as to what extent children may be allowed to suffer or even die from such a potentially harmful event without the researcher intervening. Obviously, such studies are permissible only when at least a background of routine medical and health services is provided; preferably a higher level of care, comparable to the medical sophistication of the research staff, must be provided. The usual procedure is to provide full medical care as soon as a child shows signs of severe malnutrition, but to leave the child otherwise untouched. It may be argued that even such care is too late and insufficient. Another strategy is to provide all the children in the study with some sort of care, but of different forms so that the results of the different regimes can be observed. Here, however, the situation arises that under certain regimes, children will die unless treated under another regime. Furthermore such studies assess the effects of different types of intervention but are no longer specifically geared to testing the hypothesis that malnutrition influences mental development. Whatever form of care is provided, the study will interfere with the social reality that is being studied and consequently influence it. For example, children who would otherwise have died will now stay alive; furthermore, the range of malnutrition that occurs among the children is restricted, the more severe forms being prevented or quickly treated. Whatever solutions are sought to these ethical questions, they must obviously prevail over the methodological demands and will consequently lead to various imperfections of design.

2.6 Longitudinal studies

The term longitudinal we reserve for studies in which children are examined at regular intervals before, or from, their episode of malnutrition onwards. Contrary to the usual practice in follow-up studies, the children in the different groups are selected at the time of malnutrition. However, because of the loss of subjects over the years, this does not pose an essential difference to follow-up studies. The important difference is that a longitudinal study is conceived before or at the time of the children's suffering and that data are collected throughout the years. It must be pointed out that the distinction between longitudinal and follow-up studies is in practice often less clear than when theoretically formulated. For example, a study which collects anthropometric and medical data throughout the years is a longitudinal study. If, after a number of years, it is suddenly decided to carry out psychological examinations, it is doubtful whether this psychological study could be considered longitudinal. Wall and Williams have discussed the problems that are inherent to longitudinal studies and some of their remarks follow here,

> Individuals for longitudinal study often have to be chosen in terms of their accessibility and co-operativeness, which rènders them unrepresentative and makes generalization suspect. Over long periods of time attrition of the sample occurs, and it is often difficult to state precisely the comparability of the initial and final groups. In this connection, too, we should note the objection that continued study of the same individuals carries with it the risk of modifying their behaviour in unknown ways. ...
> The passage of time leads to changes in the hypotheses and in the questions raised, and to unforeseen and unforeseeable changes in instrumentation and theory. The tendency is to start out with a comprehensive and mixed bag of variables and measures, to add to these as time goes on... .
> In the course of a longitudinal study carried on over many years, it is likely that new hypotheses will arise either from the study itself or from general advances in the relevant fields of social science. There is a reasonable chance, say the critics, that the refutation or verification of these will depend upon anterior data which were not collected because their possible significance was not perceived. (Wall and Williams, 1970, pp. 19-20.)

The great advantage of longitudinal studies is that they compile information on intellectual growth and the factors that influence its course. Such investigations, ideally, produce a view of the total constellation of factors that influence a child's mental development throughout the years. Follow-up studies may attempt to collect similar information but only afterwards, making the information far more restricted in nature and less reliable.

However, in both follow-up and longitudinal designs malnutrition is studied in its natural surroundings, and these studies are not true experiments, if only because the randomization of subjects is not possible. Theoretically, therefore, *selection* always offers an alternative explanation for any observed (or lack of observed) effects, whatever precautions the researcher may take (Campbell and Stanley, 1966; Kerlinger, 1972). Furthermore, since children are usually studied for many years, some may be lost in the process. This *attrition* also offers a potential explanation for differences or lack of differences in the case where it affects the index and the comparison children differently. The longitudinal studies can check whether this is indeed the case, while this is hardly possible with follow-up studies.

2.7 Intervention studies

Intervention studies try to achieve at least some degree of control over the independent variable of malnutrition. Although malnutrition cannot randomly be introduced among children, its occurrence can be prevented through food supplementation among some children and left to (partly) take its natural course among other children. However, the allocation to conditions can never be completely random. Usually the supplementation will be provided on a voluntary basis, which necessarily leads to selection within this group, in this case not so much of children who suffer from malnutrition but of children who are regularly supplemented. In fact, one large-scale intervention study in Guatemala was conceived on the assumption that of the 350 children at the start of the study, over a period of 7 years only 10% would continuously have sought supplementation and thus qualify as an experimental group (Habicht, Yarbrough, and Klein, 1974, p. 36). On the other hand, in the non-supplemented group, not all the children will fall prey to malnutrition, but only those who would have suffered from it naturally, which again introduces selection. Although in large-scale studies the degree and the importance of the selection that occurs within the supplemented and non-supplemented groups can be observed, if it occurs (and one is never quite sure why it occurs), it is difficult, if not impossible, to handle (Tuddenham, 1974, p. 76).

Theoretically, several intervention designs can be drawn up, but in practice only two types of study are feasible, one in which the family, the other in which the village or community, is used as the unit of supplementation. Clearly, over long periods, it is impossible to make food available for one child in a family, and to expect the mother not to give any of this food to her other children. Apart from the problems this would create within the families concerned, the distinction between supplemented and non-supplemented children could easily be blurred. Supplementation must at least be given to all children in one family. Comparisons can then be made with siblings who grew up before the supplementation was introduced and with children from non-supplemented families.

Supplementing the children in one family but not those in a neighbouring family may also raise difficulties. In fact, several authors are of the opinion that completely random supplementation *within* one community is not feasible (Billewicz, 1974b, p. 58; Tuddenham, 1974, p. 79). For this reason, some researchers prefer a design in which communities as a whole receive supplementation and other comparable communities do not, which reduces the chance of contamination of the different experimental groups. A major problem with this design lies in the finding of communities that are identical in all relevant aspects, perhaps an impossible task. Furthermore, the intervention study may decide the absence of malnutrition but little more. When the effects of different patterns of malnutrition must be studied, the researcher cannot induce a certain type of malnutrition in one group and another type in a second group. Instead, he has to depend upon the natural occurrence of these different patterns of malnutrition, just as in longitudinal and follow-up studies.

Also, intervention studies, strictly speaking, do not test the hypothesis that malnutrition interferes with intellectual development; rather they test the hypothesis that intervention has a positive effect on intellectual abilities. Even when the latter turns out to be the case, the conclusion that malnutrition has a negative effect is logically not warranted. Although this may appear a somewhat academic point, it is not. As long as it is not convincingly shown by what avenues the intervention influences intellectual development, it may well be that aspects other than nutrition *per se* have led to the improvement. The attention necessarily given to the target group is potentially a distorting factor, the more so the longer the period of observation. Certain aspects of this attention, such as the effects of repeated testing, can be controlled for with manipulation of designs, but other, subtler changes may also occur, e.g. in expectancy and motivation in the individual or the community. These, in their turn, may influence the child's development. Thus looms a confounding variable, similar to those met in follow-up and longitudinal studies. Another source of invalidity, as pointed out by Campbell and Stanley (1966) is that of interaction between selection and treatment. Those mothers who continuously seek supplementation are probably a very select group, and the possibility cannot be excluded that the supplementation falls here on particularly fertile ground.

The conclusion of this discussion must be that in regard to questions of causality, all the research designs that have been discussed are less than perfect. Warren's assertion (1973) that the only relevant investigations in this field are the longitudinal and intervention studies currently being carried out in South and Middle America (Canosa, 1968; Cravioto, Birch, DeLicardie, Rosales, and Vega, 1969; Latham and Cobos, 1971) is, on the one hand, unduly strict in its methodological demands and, on the other, overly optimistic in its expectations of these studies. It is by means of the judicious use of different research designs and different comparison groups in the investigation of more and more specific research questions that insight will be gained. Another critic is even more pessimistic and doubts whether inquiries along these lines will get us much further since no definite answers can be provided (Tizard, 1974b, p. 69). These critics overlook one maxim of hypothetical-deductive models of knowledge collection, namely, that theories (and also hypotheses) are not confirmed or proven. Instead they are exposed to falsification and may fail to be rejected. If falsified, they may be rejected or amended. Looked at in this way, the fundamental requirement of research is not that it proves a theory or hypothesis but that these are given a fair chance to be falsified. Consequently, it is only the accumulation of successive study results that leads to a common opinion among researchers, although absolute proof for a theory or hypothesis is never given (Campbell and Stanley 1966, p. 35).

Until now we have been concerned with questions of control and design; and indeed most investigators in this field have been preoccupied, if not obsessed, with these matters, often taking for granted the instruments i.e. the tests, used. However, for most countries in those parts of the world where malnutrition is endemic – South America, Asia, and Africa – where psychological tests have been adapted or constructed, they have seldom been standardized. For example, in one study, otherwise well designed, previously malnourished Jamaican children between 5 and 11 years of age were tested with the W.I.S.C., but 20-30% of these children failed to pass any *one* item (Hertzig, Birch, Richardson, and Tizard, 1972). In other words they failed all the items of all the subtests; apparently the test was unsuited to these children.[6] Since objections are sometimes raised against the use of psychological tests in non-western societies, the instruments that are employed require discussion and careful analysis. We will first briefly review the relevant experiences of psychological testing in Africa in the next chapter.

3. The Testing of Intellectual Abilities in Africa

The testing of intellectual abilities in Africa, south of the Sahara,[7] has a longer history than is generally realized. The first psychometric studies date from the turn of the century, and for a long time the testing of aptitudes and abilities was the overriding interest of psychologists in Africa (see Hoorweg and Marais, 1969). The test scores of African groups in general fell below the scores of European groups (Cryns, 1962; Faverge and Falmagne, 1962), particularly on speed tests (Ombredane, Bertelson, and Beniest-Noirot, 1958). In one of the first reviews of psychological research in Africa Doob concluded that 'the mean intelligence of samples of Africans as measured by a conventional European intelligence test, is always below that of the corresponding European norm.' (Doob, 1965, p. 382.)

In discussing this difference in test performance, authors often take a defensive position, maintaining that Africans are not genetically inferior, in whatever ability is under discussion. Instead, they attribute these differences to environmental factors. Most Africans are unfamiliar with test situations and in doubt as to what is expected of them, which affects their motivation and test strategy. This, however, is not enough to explain the full magnitude of the differences. African schoolboys who are familiar with test situations are nevertheless in general below European schoolboys in test performance. Most authors go on to argue that although, in principle, scores on intelligence tests are meant to be independent of experience, in fact they are not. European children have more training in the skills required in ability tests by their exposure to toys, pictorial and reading material, and formal education.

Inherent in the above arguments is the premise that intelligence can be quantitatively compared across cultures; that all men have some of it – some more, some less, for various reasons. This premise is rejected by others who are of the opinion that the cognitive processes of Africans differ qualitatively from those of Europeans, and that quantitative comparisons are futile. The question whether fundamental differences in thought processes accompany cultural differences has been the subject of a prolonged debate among opposing anthropological schools,

> ... one school of thought maintains that salient differences in beliefs and category systems represent no more than differing conventions with little impact on thought processes; the opposing school holds that *either* a difference in beliefs *or* a difference in classification systems is sufficient evidence for differing thought processes. (Cole, Gay, Glick, and Sharp, 1971, p. 3.)

In recent years, psychologists have also contributed to this argument by studying the cognitive development of children in different cultures. The theories of Piaget about the basic structures and functioning of higher mental processes, which do lend themselves to use in different cultures, have stimulated a considerable amount of research (Dasen, 1972). The studies in Africa indicate that the sequence of cognitive stages in African children is not different from that in European children, but that schooling is of utmost importance. Formal education not only decides when operations are mastered, but also whether certain operations are mastered at all. As regards a qualitative difference in thought processes between different cultural groups, Cole and Scribner, after reviewing the evidence, argue that,

> ... we are unlikely to find cultural differences in basic component cognitive processes. While we cannot completely rule out this possibility, there is no evidence, in any line of investigation that we have reviewed, that any cultural

group wholly lacks a basic process such as abstraction, or inferential reasoning, or categorization. (Cole and Scribner, 1974, p. 193.)

Whatever the position on this issue, it would be wrong to conclude that there is no need or use for research with standard, western-type intelligence tests in Africa. Vernon has pointed out that there is every reason 'for using such tests to study the effects of extreme environmental differences on intellectual and educational development.' (Vernon, 1969a, p. 76.) They are also useful in studying educational and vocational success, and for obvious, practical reasons, the development of test batteries for selection purposes in Africa has usually consisted of the adaptation of standard tests. Some of the material that has been gathered in such studies also provides insight into the structure of abilities of Africans.

3.1 The structure of African abilities

The first relevant studies were those carried out among army recruits in East Africa and among mining recruits in South Africa. Already some time before 1945, MacDonald[8] gave a battery of tests, including dexterity tests, mechanical tests, formboards, a block design test, two matrices tests, and an arithmetic test to between 1000 and 1850 army recruits. Centroid factor analysis yielded a three-factor structure, which was left unrotated. In 1950, Vernon, in *The Structure of Human Abilities*, published the results of the same battery of tests with between 308 and 631 recruits. Again three unrotated factors were extracted, but the author discarded the third. The first factor could not be interpreted as 'g' or 'educing relations' since it gave high loadings with the formboard and dexterity tests. However, the author regarded the second factor as 'the cognitive factor ... quite close to British g, while the opposite pole is a mixture of our manual dexterity and physical factors.' (Vernon, 1971, p. 106.)

Similar efforts took place in South Africa in the mining industry. Biesheuvel (1952) developed a battery of performance tests for the selection of African mining recruits. The final battery is known as the G(eneral) A(daptability) B(attery). Factor analysis of the tests in the battery resulted in one general factor which was interpreted as 'practical general intelligence' (Biesheuvel, 1954). Grant and Schepers (1969) contest that African intelligence is characterized by such a simple structure and argue that the unity of structure was a result of the few and the relatively unsophisticated tests that were used. These authors reanalysed Vernon's (previously mentioned) results and rotated the two dimensions to produce a 'dexterity' factor and a second factor 'eduction of relations'. The last factor is composed primarily of the arithmetic test, matrices, and block design. Next the authors concentrated on the G.A.B., adding five new tests and giving this battery to a group of 90 African mining recruits. After factor analysis, two factors resulted, the first, 'eduction of relations', the second, 'speed of perception'. There were also indications of a 'spatial' factor which Grant (1970) further explored. The G.A.B. and four new spatial tests were given to 100 recruit mineworkers. The spatial tests indeed produced a distinct factor which the author recognizes as 'visualization', while the original G.A.B. is again characterized as 'speed of perception'. In a further study with literate and illiterate Venda adults, residing in urban and rural areas, a battery of performance tests resulted in five factors: a 'perceptual speed' factor, a 'perceptual analysis' factor, a 'perception of form relations' factor, a 'conceptual reasoning' factor, and a 'space' factor (Grant, 1972, p. 394).

All these factor analytic studies have relied upon performance tests, tests that avoid verbal questions and answers. Anastasi points out that

> ... it cannot be assumed that nonverbal tests measure the same functions as verbal tests, however similar they may appear. A spatial analogies test is not merely a nonverbal version of a verbal analogies test. Some of the early nonlanguage tests, such as the Army Beta, were heavily loaded with spatial visualization and perceptual abilities, which are quite unrelated to verbal and numerical abilities. Even in tests like the Progressive Matrices and other nonlanguage

> tests deliberately designed to tap reasoning and abstract conceptualization, factorial analyses have revealed a large contribution of nonverbal factors to the variance of test scores. (Anastasi, 1968, p. 252.)

One wonders to what extent the previous studies have been limited to investigating spatial-perceptual abilities.

This limitation does not apply to a series of studies of school pupils in East and Central Africa. Irvine (1969a) brings this material together, reanalysing previous studies and presenting five new ones. Two of the studies were made with 700 and 1600 African students upon completion of 8 years of education, in Zambia and Rhodesia, respectively. Other studies were carried out among 70 pupils at a Zambian mining school, again with 8 years primary education, and among 400 Zambian students with 10 years of education. One study took place at a Kenyan secondary school with 180 boys having 10 to 12 years of education. The tests used in these studies varied, but some of them were employed in more than one instance. In at least three of the studies the results of the examination papers were included in the analysis. In each study, the analysis resulted in four dimensions that underly the scores on individual tests. As regards the first two studies, Irvine interprets the first factor as 'verbal-educational', the second as 'number-educational', and the third as 'g'. 'V-educational' consists of two English papers and several verbal tests (vocabulary, spelling, comprehension). 'N-educational' consists of a computation test and arithmetic papers. 'G' is loaded by the Raven-matrices and a test for abstraction. Irvine is satisfied that in the other studies, similar structures of 'g', 'v-educational' and 'n-educational' are present. Upon closer inspection, this conclusion appears unwarranted. Although the presence of 'verbal-educational' and 'number-educational' factors is fairly well established and constant over studies, this is different for 'g'. Irvine labels that factor 'g', or 'general reasoning', on which the Raven-matrices loads highest but disregards the loadings of other tests. While in the first two studies, 'g' consists of Raven-matrices and two verbal tests, in the next study (at the Zambian mining school) the Raven-matrices does not combine with these two tests but with another test, A.I.R. (boxes and mechanical), although not with the A.I.R. figures. In the next Zambian study, the Raven-matrices combines with A.I.R. boxes and figures, but not with A.I.R. mechanical or vocabulary. Reanalysing two previous studies, Irvine finds that in one study the Raven-matrices constitutes one factor with a block design test and an arithmetic test. In the other study two reasoning factors and one perceptual factor are found. Vernon cautions that, 'The role of factor analysis in the study of individual or group differences should not be exaggerated. Primarily it is a formal scheme for classifying and interpreting test performances, and should not be considered as a means to identifying the basic abilities of human beings.' (Vernon, 1969b, p. 22.) That the tests group themselves differently in the studies that are discussed must, without doubt, be attributed partly to the fact that different test batteries were used in the different studies. The existence of 'g', or a 'general reasoning' factor, stands in need of further study. One can agree with Irvine's cautious summary that '...when Western-based tests purporting to identify abilities are used, they will generally reproduce the same theoretical dimensions in other cultures, although the contributions of individual tests are by no means constant.' (Irvine, 1974, p. 249.)

Vernon (1969a) carried out a series of studies of boys between the ages of 10 and 12 years in England, the Hebrides, Jamaica, Uganda and Canada (Eskimo and Indian children), using varying test batteries. In all the studies four factors emerged which the author designates as 'g', 'verbal-educational', 'spatial', and 'drawing'. In three studies these factors also emerged in this order, but the results of the other studies differ in respect of the dominance of the 'g' and the 'verbal-educational' factors. Among Canadian Indians these two dimensions show very similar test loadings, while in the Hebrides study they merged into one factor. Among the Ugandan group the first factor was a 'verbal-educational' one and the second is called 'general reasoning'. The impression that the existence of 'g' is problematical remains, although its existence cannot be excluded either. The separate 'drawing' factor that is reported results from the fact that several drawing tests were included.

In summary it can be said first that meaningful research has been carried out with standard-type psychological tests in Africa. Secondly, that, depending upon the tests used and the populations studied, these tests may arrange themselves in 'spatial-perceptual' and 'verbal/numerical-educational' groups. If a 'general reasoning' or 'g' group exists, it appears to be relatively unstable.

4. Objectives and Design of the Study

From 1953 until 1973 the British Medical Research Council operated a child nutrition research unit in Kampala, Uganda. The first director of the unit was Dr. R.F.A. Dean. Up to 1962 some 1000 patients were treated here. Most of the acutely malnourished children admitted to this clinic were first seen at a rural clinic at Namulonge, some 19 km from Kampala. Healthy children were also regularly seen during their early years at the Namulonge clinic. Many of the children were occasionally seen throughout their later years and the records of all children were carefully preserved with the idea of follow-up studies later on.

The present study availed itself of these records and has the following research objectives. The primary objectives were to investigate:

1. the long-term effect of malnutrition on intellectual and motor abilities,
2. the influence of the age at which malnutrition occurs,
3. the influence of the type and severity of the malnutrition, and
4. the nature of the effect.

The secondary objectives of the study were:

1. to look for any signs among the previously malnourished children of their catching up in terms of intellectual abilities between the ages of 11 and 17 years, and
2. to collect information regarding their daily behaviour.

4.1 Design

Three groups of 20 children (to be called *index* children) who had been admitted for protein-energy malnutrition to the Kampala clinic were selected. The age at admission for children in group 1 was between 8 and 15 months, for group 2 between 16 and 21 months, and for group 3 between 22 and 27 months. A comparison group of 20 children (group 4), who had not suffered from acute malnutrition, was selected from those who had attended the rural clinic at Namulonge. The comparison children had been weighed at frequent intervals over a period of at least two years starting in the first year of life. Comparison children were selected only if during this period their weights had not fallen below the tenth percentile of the weight figures given by Stuart and Stevenson (1954) for children of north European descent. Two comparison children fell below the tenth percentile on one occasion each, but notes made at the time did not record any clinical signs of malnutrition.

A randomized block design (Brownlee, 1965; Winer, 1971) was used in which the four groups of children were individually matched. For each child one comparison child in each of the other groups was found, forming a block of four children who matched each other. To eliminate any variations due to tribal differences, it was decided that only Baganda children would be studied.

The actual selection procedure was as follows. The records of all Baganda children who had been admitted to the clinic before 27 months of age and who were now between 11 and 17 years of age were taken from the files. The children were then arranged into the three respective malnourished groups: admitted before 15 months of age, between 16 and 21 months, and between 22 and 27 months of age. In Buganda malnutrition at one year of age has always been less frequent than later malnutrition, and the first group therefore had the smallest number of children. Once a child in this group had been located, a number of children of the same sex and age in the other two malnourished groups were selected from the records, and efforts were made to find them. Likewise for the comparison children. Once several of these children had been found, an appropriate 'match' was selected in each group and further efforts to locate the other children were discontinued.

Records of the tracing were kept for the first malnourished group (group 1) and the comparison children (group 4). As far as the first group is concerned, attempts were made to locate 32 children; 29 of these children were found and 2 were not, while the last case had moved too far away to be visited. Thus 3 children (9%) were not found. As regards the comparison group, attempts were made to locate 58 children. Of these children, 52 were found, 20 of whom constitute the comparison group (group 4). Two children could not be found and the attempts to locate the remaining 4 children were stopped because they were no longer needed. Thus 6 children (10%) out of 58 were not found. The families of the children who could not be located usually had moved to another village or town where the trail could not be picked up again, although they were not the only families that had moved. In this respect, a failure rate of only 10% is low. The success of the tracing must be attributed to the competence and perseverance of our assistants, Mr. Semindi and Mr. Mukasa, the two elderly Baganda who had sufficient experience and social standing to command respect and to be able to request information throughout Buganda. Moreover, in a society like this, which is by and large traditional, people usually live near relatives who are often able to provide information about those who have moved away. Since we are dealing with small numbers of subjects, it is very unlikely that the 10% of children who were not found (3 and 6 children, respectively) will have resulted in bias.

The child's date of birth was checked against the village birth registers when necessary, and any doubt or discrepancy about the date of birth excluded a child from the study. Children with any history signifying possible brain insult, such as convulsions or respiratory infections with anoxia were excluded, as were those with long-term chronic infections such as tuberculosis. Severe anaemia did not exclude a child unless a disturbance of consciousness or convulsions were recorded.

From among the children in groups 2, 3, and 4 who had been located, in each group that child was selected as a 'match' who was nearest to a child in group 1: first in sex, age, and education, and secondly as regards the education of the parents and the general socio-economic status of their families as reflected by material possessions.

Since we could not avail ourselves beforehand of any valid indicators of socio-economic status, information on a wide range of material possessions was collected for each family either through observation or questioning. No information was sought which might have proved embarrassing to collect or impossible to ascertain with precision, such as money income or farm acreage. Analysis of these data was carried out for a group of 30 children, consisting of the 20 comparison children in group 4 and 10 more children (group 5) for whom further particulars are given in chapter 5 (p. 54). Items which were either absent or present in all or most households were laid aside. Correlational analysis and Guttman scaling of the remaining items resulted in two scales. The first is composed mainly of modern household and luxury items which would have demanded a cash outlay: type and condition of the house, and the presence of a table, arm-chairs, a radio, a gramophone, and a car (see appendix G). This scale is referred to as *modern expenditure*. For the 60 previously malnourished children in groups 1, 2, and 3 the coefficient of reproducibility of this scale was .90 and the coefficient of scalability .56. The second scale consists mainly of the traditional economic resources that a family may have at its disposal: plots of land, the number of cows owned, of workers employed, and of rooms in the house, and, oddly, the possession of a bicycle (see appendix G). This scale is called *traditional resources*, and has a reproducibility coefficient of .89 and a scalability coefficient of .49 for the 60 malnourished children. 'Traditional resources' and 'modern expenditure' are not unrelated and correlate significantly (.37). This socio-economic information was also available for 76 children who had been traced but not included in the study. For this group of children the reproducibility coefficient of both scales was .90, while the coefficients of scalability were .57 and .48, respectively. The correlation between the two scales was again .37.

The results of the matching are presented in table 2, and the age, sex, and education of each child are listed in appendix A.

Table 2 *Study design: environmental variables (means and standard deviations)*

	Malnourished children, age on admission: 8-15 months	16-21 months	22-27 months	Comparison group
Group number	1	2	3	4
	N = 20	N = 20	N = 20	N = 20
Boys	11	11	11	11
Girls	9	9	9	9
Child: present age (years)	14.1 *(S.D. = 1.3)*	14.0 *(1.5)*	13.8 *(1.4)*	13.9 *(1.5)*
Child: education (years)	4.6 *(1.6)*	4.5 *(1.3)*	4.4 *(1.2)*	4.4 *(1.4)*
Male Guardian: education (years)	3.1 *(3.3)*	5.4 *(2.5)*	4.9 *(3.3)*	5.7 *(3.0)*
Female Guardian: education (years)	3.2 *(2.8)*	3.6 *(2.5)*	1.4 *(2.3)*	3.5 *(2.1)*
Socio-Economic Status: modern expenditure	3.6 *(2.2)*	2.6 *(1.2)*	2.3 *(1.7)*	2.7 *(2.4)*
trad. resources	2.7 *(1.7)*	2.2 *(0.9)*	1.8 *(1.1)*	1.9 *(1.6)*

The sex composition of the groups is identical, as are, for all practical purposes, the age and education of the groups. The average age of the children is 14 years, and they have, on average, attended 4.5 years of formal education. Although there are differences between the groups regarding the education of the parents and the socio-economic status of the families, these differences do not consistently favour one group. The comparison group scores highest on only one variable (that is, the education of the father), closely followed by one of the malnourished groups. For the other three variables it is always one of the malnourished groups which achieves the highest score. Since the main objective of the matching is to insure that the social background of the comparison children does not differ from that of the previously malnourished children, an analysis of variance (one-way) was carried out, as a check, for the last four variables. A contrast of the comparison group with the three malnourished groups reveals that the small differences that do exist are not significant and that they also go both ways. The three malnourished groups among themselves show slightly larger differences. The education of the male guardian is lowest in group 1, but the education of the female guardian is lowest in group 3. This group is also lowest on the two socio-economic scales suggesting that it is perhaps slightly less well off than groups 1 and 2, although the education of the male guardian is lowest in group 1. As we will see, group 3 is not used on its own when the different malnourished groups are compared, but it is combined with group 2. Because the average level of education of both parents is highest in group 2, combining groups 2 and 3 compensates for the slight possibility that the children in group 3 have a background that is somewhat lower in socio-economic status.

As described in the previous chapter there are indications that, at least in Uganda, family stability is related to the occurrence of malnutrition. Conceivably, family stability is also an important factor in the intellectual development of children. Although not purposely matched on this characteristic, the four groups are nevertheless not different in respect of the present family situation of the children (table 3). Only 15-25% of the children are living with both parents, 45-55% live with either father or mother, while 25-35% are living with persons other than their parents. The incidence of divorce in Buganda is known to be very high (Mair, 1934; Fallers, 1960; Southwold, 1965).

4.2 Components of malnutrition: the condition of the malnourished children during their admission 10 to 16 years previously (1954–61)

The admission records contained data about the type and severity of the malnutrition of each child. From these data seven important indicators of the condition of each child at admission were selected.

Most children lost some weight immediately after admission, mainly as a result of loss of oedema. This initial weight loss was expressed as a percentage of the weight after admission. The lowest weight recorded for the child during its stay in the unit was expressed as a percentage of the expected weight for the age of the child, using Baganda standards. These Baganda standards consist of the mean weights of healthy Baganda children as reported by Rutishauser (1965). The lowest hæmoglobin level during admission and the serum protein level at admission were recorded in grams per 100 ml. Oedema and overall clinical severity had been rated from 1 to 5 (severe), and skin changes

Table 3. *Present family situation of children*

	Malnourished children, age on admission: 8-15 months	16-21 months	22-27 months	Comparison Group
Group number	1	2	3	4
living with both parents	25%	15%	20%	25%
living with father or mother	45%	55%	45%	45%
living with neither parent	25%	25%	30%	30%
married, living with husband	1 (5%)	1 (5%)	1 (5%)	–

Table 4 *Condition of index children at admission (N = 60)*

	Mean	Standard deviation
percentage of expected weight for age [a,b]	69.7%	9.7
percentage of weight lost after admission	8.4%	6.1
hæmoglobin level [b]	6.7 g	2.1
serum protein level	4.2 g	0.7
oedema [d]	3.8	0.8
skin changes [e]	2.7	1.0
overall clinical severity [c,d]	3.3	0.9

(a) Baganda standards (Dean, 1954; Rutishauser, 1965).
(b) lowest level during hospitalization.
(c) as judged by the attending doctor.
(d) rated on ordinal scale ranging from 1 to 5 (severe).
(e) rated on ordinal scale ranging from 1 to 4 (severe).

from 1 to 4 (severe) on an ordinal scale by the doctor present at the time of admission.

The results of the examinations of the index children are presented in table 4, and the individual data for each child are presented in appendix B. After being admitted to the ward these children, on average, lost 8.4% of their weight. The lowest recorded weight of the index children was, on average, only 0.7 times the Baganda mean weight. None of these children was above 0.9 times this standard, and only seven children remained above 0.8 times this standard. As mentioned, the requirement for the comparison children was that their weights had not fallen below the (Boston) tenth percentile, which means that, during the period of observation, their weights had stayed well above 0.9 times the mean weight of healthy Baganda children. The biochemical tests revealed that serum protein of the index children averaged 4.2 g per 100 ml which falls considerably below normal values. Hæmoglobin levels on admission were also low: on average 6.7 g per 100 ml. No biochemical tests had been taken for the comparison children. The index children at admission also showed other signs of malnutrition which had not been seen in the comparison children. Some degree of oedema, ranging from mild to severe, was present in all the children, and skin changes were observed in 87% of the children.

For each of the three malnourished groups, the correlations between these seven indicators were computed. The three resulting correlation matrices were pooled in one matrix, which was subjected to principal component analysis. The main objective of principal component analysis (and of factor analysis) is to attain as systematic and economic a description of observed data as possible. The complex relationships existing among the observed data are expressed as the relation between each variable and a few underlying dimensions. This analysis, in this case, yielded two independent dimensions of malnutrition (table 5), that were to a greater or lesser extent present in each child.

Table 5 *Medical indicators at admission: varimax rotation of first two principal components (malnourished groups pooled; N = 3 x 20)*

	dimension 1	dimension 2
percentage of expected weight for age [a,b]	.07	–.80
percentage of weight lost after admission	.58	–.55
hæmoglobin level [b]	–.28	–.66
serum protein level	–.59	–.10
oedema	.73	–.17
skin changes	.69	.00
overall clinical severity [c]	.73	.23

(a) Baganda standards (Dean, 1954; Rutishauser, 1965)
(b) lowest level during hospitalization.
(c) as judged by the attending doctor.

The first dimension is composed of those variables which are predominant in kwashiorkor, that is metabolic abnormality (low serum protein levels giving rise to the oedema and initial weight loss during treatment after admission) and skin changes. The doctor's judgement of severity on admission appears to vary mainly with the degree of this dimension. The dominant element in the second dimension is the weight deficit characteristic of marasmus, with stunting of growth. Hæmoglobin deficit also loads highly on this component.

The condition of each child at admission can be described in terms of these two dimensions. We have chosen to call these components 'acute malnutrition' and 'chronic undernutrition' instead of kwashiorkor and marasmus, respectively, for purposes of clarity. Kwashiorkor or marasmus are used clinically as diagnostic terms for the total syndrome and it would be confusing to apply them to describe its components. Furthermore, the variables in each of the two dimensions tend to evolve over different periods of time (as described in chapter 2, p. 19). The first dimension is composed of acute changes developing usually over a short time and often precipitating the admission to the hospital. The second, consisting of weight deficit and hæmoglobin deficit, generally requires some period of time to develop and thus reflects the chronic nature of the malnutrition. Loss of weight after admission is related to both components but in opposite directions. Initial loss of weight during early treatment is characteristic of the acute condition. The less the weight loss, the less severe is the acute condition and the more severe is the chronic nature of the malnutrition.

For each child the severity of these two components, *'acute*

Table 6 *Average severity of 'acute malnutrition' and 'chronic undernutrition' in the three malnourished groups at admission (positive = severe)*

	group 1	group 2	group 3
'Acute malnutrition'	–.28	–.09	.20
'Chronic undernutrition'	.36	–.10	–.23

malnutrition' and *'chronic undernutrition'*, was computed as a weighted index, with a standard deviation of 1.0, of the scores on the original seven variables (principal component analysis permits the direct calculation of these weights). The severity of the 'acute malnutrition' is slightly higher in the groups admitted at a later age, while 'chronic undernutrition' is slightly more severe in the younger children (table 6). These differences are in the expected direction but far from significant.

4.3 Examinations during the present study (1970-71)

The examination of each child commenced with the psychological examination at the child's home. The test situation was kept standard by using a converted Volkswagen bus that was driven to the child's home. The second part of the examination took place some days later. On this occasion the child was collected from home, and a routine medical examination was performed at the clinic by the paediatrician on the team (J.P.S.) who concluded the session with an examination of motor development. During this visit, anthropometric measurements were also taken.

4.4 Medical examination

To ensure that at the time of testing the different groups of children were in a similar state of health, a clinical examination of all the children was conducted which revealed no serious disease. One child had an acute pyomyositis, which delayed the assessment of motor development for two weeks. The spleen was palpable in 11 of the children, scattered among all four groups. There was a considerable amount of tineal skin infection with resulting slight lymphadenopathy. Two children had an old poliomyelitis, one involving the right shoulder and arm, and the other the right leg. Hæmoglobin and serum protein levels were all within normal limits, and the mean values were similar in all four groups. An estimate of the stage of each child's puberty was attempted and the scatter from prepubertal to postpubertal was similar in the four groups. Two of the eldest girls in the previously malnourished groups were pregnant, and one in the comparison group was nursing a three-month-old baby.

4.5 Anthropometry

The senior nutritionist at the Medical Research Council Unit measured height, weight, head- and mid-upper-arm circumference, triceps skinfold- and subscapular skinfold-thickness, and interiliac diameter using standard anthropometric techniques and equipment. An X-ray of hand and wrist was also taken. The results of the anthropometric investigation have been published elsewhere (Hoorweg and Stanfield, 1976). The previously malnourished children (groups 1-3) are significantly below the comparison children (group 4) in height, weight, and head circumference, but mid-upper-arm circumference, skin-fold thicknesses, and interiliac diameter are not significantly different. There are also no significant differences in bone maturation and osteoperosis (Briers, Hoorweg and Stanfield, 1975). There are no differences of any importance among the three malnourished groups themselves.

Reduced growth as reflected by height and head circumference have widely been reported to result from malnutrition (see Habicht, Martorell, Yarbrough, Malina, and Klein, 1974). The absence of any significant differences on the other anthropometric measurements indicates that the present nutritional status of the four groups is not different. The average ratio between the present actual weight and the weight that could be expected for the height does not fall below 100% in any of the four groups. This indicates, disregarding the stunting of growth, that the present nutritional status of the children is satisfactory.

5. The Construction and the Adaptation of Tests

In the present study a general reasoning test, a verbal test, a numerical test, and three spatial-perceptual tests were included. Furthermore, three tests for short-term memory, rote learning, and incidental learning were selected because findings elsewhere indicated that memory processes might be particularly affected in malnourished children (Klein *et al.*, 1969). Motor ability was also examined, while interviews with the parents inquired about the day-to-day behaviour of the child. This chapter is concerned with the first nine tests, while motor ability and daily behaviour will be discussed in separate chapters.

The tests were first tried out on a pilot group of 18 pupils attending a rural primary school with a mean age of 12.2 years and a mean education of 5.8 years. This served to signal and eliminate problems with test instructions or test content. For some tests, a first selection of items was made after this stage.

Comprehensive construction and validation of tests for the Baganda children, to which the study was limited, would have been far too time-consuming. Therefore, the data to be used in test construction and the data needed for hypothesis testing were collected simultaneously. All the tests were given in their full, initial versions to all 80 children in the three different malnourished groups (1, 2, and 3) and the comparison group (4). The final adaptation of the standard tests and the final construction of newly developed tests consisted of selecting reliable items and developing adequate scoring systems. These calculations were carried out on the basis of the data collected for the

20 comparison children (group 4) and for 10 more children (group 5). These 10 children also had not been malnourished in early childhood, and they fulfil similar requirements to the comparison children in group 4. They are of similar age, sex, education, and socio-economic background and play no further role in the study.[9] Test construction and validation relied exclusively upon the data collected for the 30 children in groups 4 and 5.

The adaptations introduced in the standard tests are discussed separately for each test and are summarized in table 7. For all tests a comprehensive standard instruction was given, while for some tests extra practice was allowed. The tests were all given individually and did not rely upon written instructions or written questions. They were all conducted in the children's tongue, Luganda, with the help of a female interpreter. Because African children are particularly at a disadvantage with speed tests, speed bonuses were abolished for all tests. However, to keep children from lingering too long on a single item, the time limits were not abolished, but doubled.

Some of the tests in this battery rely heavily upon the use of colours. Therefore, all children were first examined with the tests developed by Ishihara (1959). Not a single case of colour blindness was encountered.

5.1 General reasoning

The Raven-matrices is generally considered the best available measure of general reasoning or 'g' (Savage, 1968). In this test, master designs which have a part missing are presented. Out of six smaller patterns, that one which completes the master design must be chosen. Considerable experience has been gained with this test in Africa. The order of item difficulty may vary with different cultures, and performance on the test improves with experience and education (Anastasi, 1968; Irvine, 1969; Wober, 1969). In this study, the coloured matrices (Raven, 1965) were used. During the pilot trials, we found that most children adopted quite early an incorrect answering strategy. At these moments, the children usually seemed unsure as to what to do and

Table 7 *Modifications in standard tests*

	Items	Introduction and examination	Scoring and time limits	Miscellaneous
Raven-coloured-matrices	34 out of 36.	First error of each series: question, 'are you quite sure?'.	x	Board form.
Arithmetic (WISC)	15 out of 16. Items 14 and 15 simplified.	x	No time bonuses. Time limits doubled.	Items 14 and 15 presented verbally.
Porteus-mazes	5 out of 12.	x	No time bonuses	x
Block-design (WAIS)	x	2 extra introductory items. First error: question, 'are you quite sure?'.	No time bonuses. Time limits doubled.	Discontinued after 2 consecutive failures.
Memory-for-designs	x	x	x	x
Knox-cubes	4 series: 2 quick, 2 slow.	x	x	x

often asked for a feedback, but when this was withheld they often decided upon a simple, incorrect answering strategy. To provide such feedback in a standard manner the boardform of the test was introduced. Here the child is presented with six pieces of wood on which the different patterns are pasted. The child must choose the correct piece and physically fit this into the master design, so that he can observe the result. To increase feedback even more, after the first error in each of the three series the child was asked, 'Are you quite sure?'. The child was then allowed to correct the answer but the item was scored as an error. On other items, one spontaneous correction was allowed. Analysis of the 30 children showed that two items (A8 and AB5) did not correlate with the total score (–.03 and –.04 respectively). They were left out of the final version, so that 34 items comprise the Raven-matrices.

5.2 Verbal ability

Vocabularies have been used among African children but usually in a foreign language (English, French) or an almost literal translation into an African language. A vocabulary in a foreign tongue will measure little more than scholastic achievement in that language. It is doubtful whether the translation of an existing vocabulary produces a more satisfactory instrument. The subtlety of synonyms and the complexity of concepts on which such tests rely tend to be culture specific and difficult, if not impossible, to transpose into another language. In using a vocabulary, a vernacular version consisting of local concepts, expressions, and equivalents is preferable.

A list of sixty Luganda words was drawn up with the help of a professional interpreter and a Baganda student in psychology. Luganda, like most African languages, abounds in metaphoric expressions. For this reason, we saw fit also to select 15 idiomatic expressions and 11 proverbs. After the pilot testing with the 18 primary school pupils, the list was reduced to 25 words and 10 idiomatic expressions, while the proverbs were omitted because the children showed themselves completely unfamiliar with these. On the basis of the p-values and item-total correlations for the 30 children in groups 4 and 5, the vocabulary was again reduced. The final version consists of 13 words and 8 idiomatic expressions, as listed in table 8. There are no indications that words and idioms constitute separate tests. Factor analysis of the 21 items over the 30 children resulted in one general factor, while no other coherent factors were present.

5.3 Numerical ability

The arithmetic test of the W.I.S.C. (Wechsler, 1949) was used. The problems were identical, but adapted to local conditions, and are fully presented in appendix F. Items 14 and 15 were

Table 8 *Vocabulary*

Words:		
obukowekowe	eyelash	
amansanganzira	crossroads	
akasimu	small, old hoe	
ebbuba	jealousy between husband and wife	
bongo	perket; curdled milk	
okuganiriza	to spend thriftly	
egandalo	to rest	
okukalatira	to instruct strongly	
okubaguliza	to point out	
luboni	down payment	
edigobe	mashed matooke	
olutuga	bracelet	
enkgandago	ladder	
Idiomatic expressions:	(literal meaning)	(figurative meaning)
yamugombe mu obwala	he gets the fingernails around	to arrest
okwokya omusubi	to burn the grass	to run
enkoko yagikwata mu mwa	he held the mouth of the cock	to rise early
okulya mu ndago	to eat in the voice	to sing, to cry (animal)
okukomba ku elima	to kiss the hoe	to refuse
okugula enyoni	to buy an airplane	to escape, run away
okuja omukono mungabo	to take the hand out of the shield	to die, yield (important person)
okumira omuke omusu	to breathe in fresh air	to die, be killed.

simplified and presented not on cards, but orally. Item 16 was considered too difficult and excluded. Time limits were doubled and time bonuses abolished. Calculation of item-total correlations over the 30 children in groups 4 and 5 did not lead to the omission of items.

5.4 Spatial-perceptual abilities

Three tests were selected. The Porteus-mazes (Arthur, 1947) were already employed in an early study in southern Africa (Porteus, 1937), and maze tests have been used repeatedly among Africans. The Porteus-mazes consists of twelve mazes that must be solved. Some mazes may have to be repeated as often as four times which makes the test rather time consuming. To shorten the test only five mazes (D, E, G, H, and J) were employed, apart from three introductory mazes (A, B2, and C1) that were not scored. This drastically reduced the range and variation of scores.

The block-design test and its predecessor, the Koh's-blocks, have also been widely used throughout Africa (see Lloyd, 1972). Geometric designs are presented on paper and must be copied by means of blocks with red, white, and red/white sides. In the present study the block-design test of the W.A.I.S. (Wechsler, 1955) was used. Vernon (1969a) reported that Ugandan schoolboys scored very low on this test. Therefore the two introductory items of the W.I.S.C. (Wechsler, 1949) were also included. Feedback was also increased. When the first incorrect solution was handed in, the child was asked, 'Are you quite sure?'. Time limits were doubled, no time bonuses were given, and the test was discontinued after two consecutive failures. The item-total correlations calculated over the 30 children in groups 4 and 5 did not lead to the omission of items.

The memory-for-designs test (Graham and Kendall, 1960) has been developed for the diagnosis of organic brain damage and calls for design copying and short-term memory. Simple geometric designs must be drawn from memory after they have been viewed for five seconds. Errors are scored.[10] U.S. norms for groups of brain-disordered patients are presented in the manual.

5.5 Short-term memory

The Knox-cubes test (Arthur, 1947) requires the child to copy, from memory, a sequence of taps on four wooden blocks. Klein *et al.* (1969) have suggested the use of this test in two different versions, one with a standard speed of presentation and a second with an increased speed of four taps per second. In the present study, a slow and a quick (two to three taps per second) version were both presented twice. The correlations between these four trials for the 30 children in groups 4 and 5 are presented in table 9.

If the slow and quick versions assess different psychological processes, the correlations among the two slow trials and the two quick trials should be the highest. They are .52 and .46 and fall in the middle of the range of observed correlations. Furthermore, the correlation between the first and the fourth trial, slow 1 and quick 2, should be the lowest of all. With .47 it also falls in the middle range. This does not confirm that slow and quick versions examine different aspects of short-term memory. Test-retest correlation for each of the two conditions, however, is rather low. The scores of each child on the four trials were therefore combined into one score for Knox-cubes.

5.6 Learning and incidental learning

Incidental learning may occur during a learning task when irrelevant information is memorized. A procedure was developed to

Table 9 *Knox-cubes: correlations between trials (Groups 4 and 5; N = 30)*

Order of presentation:	(1)	(2)	(3)	(4)
(1) slow 1	–			
(2) quick 1	.44	–		
(3) slow 2	.52	.28	–	
(4) quick 2	.47	.46	.61	–

Table 10 *Learning test*

COLOURS presented on	FORMS series A	FORMS series B	Associated ANIMAL
red			dog
light blue			goat
green			cow
yellow			pig
brown			cat
dark blue			chicken

assess both learning and incidental learning. The children were instructed to memorize the imaginary colours of six animals (see table 10). Colours were presented, one by one, and the child had to name the corresponding animal. Each colour was presented alternately in two geometrical forms. There were two series (A and B) of six forms each, twelve forms in all. The experimenter paid no attention whatsoever to these different forms. The two series, of six forms each, were presented four times. Before presentation, each series was shuffled, while the series themselves were presented in the fixed order A B B A A B A B. This rote learning task was quite easily mastered by most children. The 30 children in groups 4 and 5 attained 87.5% correct answers and the distribution of the raw scores was skewed. Therefore, a scaling system was developed. The eight presentations of the series were each scored 0 or 1, depending on how many correct answers were given in each series. The number of correct answers required to pass each of the 8 series was decided by Guttman scaling.

When this rote learning task was completed, the twelve forms were presented in white, and the colour of the form had to be recollected. As mentioned before, memorizing of the forms had not been requested and can be considered as a measure of incidental learning. The incidental-learning score consists of the number of forms for which the correct colour was named. The percentage of correct answers obtained by the 30 children in groups 4 and 5 differed in respect to different forms and series, but no systematic trends were found.

5.7 Reliability

Because the selection of items for the individual tests was based on their consistency as calculated for the 30 children in groups 4 and 5, the reliability estimates calculated for the same group might have been spuriously high. The estimates (K20) for the eight tests that are presented in table 11 were independently calculated for the 60 index children in groups 1, 2, and 3. As regards the learning test, here the coefficient of reproducibility is given. These estimates fall between .80 and .90 for six tests,

Table 11 *Reliability estimates (malnourished children, N = 60)*

Raven-matrices	.87 [a]
vocabulary	.74 [a]
arithmetic	.89 [a]
Porteus-mazes	.53 [b]
block-design	.86 [a]
memory-for-designs	.83 [a]
Knox-cubes	.86 [a]
learning	.89 [c]
incidental-learning	.54 [a]

(a) K20, with correction for variations in item difficulty (Horst, 1953).
(b) K20, with extension for tests with more than two categories of response (Ferguson, 1951).
(c) Guttman scale, coefficient of reproducibility.

notably Raven-matrices, arithmetic, block-design, memory-for-designs, Knox-cubes, and learning. The estimate for the vocabulary reaches .74, but for Porteus-mazes and incidental-learning they are lower. The reason for the relatively low reliability of the Porteus-mazes must be that only 5 of the original 12 items were retained. For the battery as a whole, reliabilities are quite satisfactory.

It must be borne in mind that these figures represent the reliabilities of the tests among this particular group of children, ranging in age from 11 to 17 years. Since the group is not homogeneous as regards age, this may have positively influenced the reliability estimates for some tests. Usually the reliability coefficients for tests are computed for more homogeneous age groups and thus are not directly comparable with those found here. With this reservation in mind, the few reliabilities reported by other studies in Africa follow. Biesheuvel (1952) claims split-half reliabilities for five subtests of the G.A.B. ranging evenly from .70 to .91. When the G.A.B. and five more tests were administered to 90 recruit mine workers, the reliabilities for the individual tests ranged from .70 to .90, with most tests above .80 (Grant and Schepers, 1969). In a study of spatial abilities somewhat lower reliabilities, between .60 and .70, were found for four tests given to 100 recruit mineworkers (Grant, 1970).

5.8 Validity

The validity of the respective tests was first examined by means of a principal component analysis, using the raw scores obtained from the 30 children in groups 4 and 5. This group was used because among the malnourished children, the structure of abilities may possibly have been influenced by the malnutrition. Although the data for these children were also used in test construction, this presents no difficulties because test construction was based solely on internal analysis within each test. Table 12A presents the first three dimensions after varimax rotation.[11] These three components account for 67.6% of the total variance. Component scores were calculated and the correlations of these with age, education, and sex are presented in table 12B. The first dimension is predominantly loaded by Raven-matrices, vocabulary, and arithmetic and correlates high with both age and education. When age is held constant, the resulting partial correlation of the first component with education is still .55. This component thus presents not only a general reasoning, but also an educational, dimension. The second component is identified mainly by block-design and Porteus-mazes, while memory-for-designs also loads on this dimension. It is unrelated to age or education, presenting a spatial-perceptual dimension which correlates negatively with sex, i.e. girls score

Table 12

A. Tests: varimax rotation of first three principal components (Groups 4 and 5; N = 30)

	dimension 1	dimension 2	dimension 3
Raven-matrices	.73	.15	.39
vocabulary	.83	–.12	–.22
arithmetic	.75	.37	.11
Porteus-mazes	.26	.82	–.01
block-design	–.04	.86	.19
memory-for-designs	.12	.58	.46
Knox-cubes	.04	.36	.64
learning	.31	.32	.57
incidental-learning	–.09	–.09	.87

B. Correlations of three principal components with age, education and sex (Groups 4 and 5; N = 30)

	dimension 1	dimension 2	dimension 3
age	.65	–.15	.12
education	.76	–.02	.18
sex	–.02	–.54	.36

Table 13 *Tests: three principal components after statistical removal of age differences (Groups 4 and 5; N = 30)*

	dimension 1	dimension 2	dimension 3
Raven-matrices	.65	.19	.42
vocabulary	.77	–.13	–.31
arithmetic	.66	.39	.09
Porteus-mazes	.14	.86	–.04
block-design	.09	.84	.22
memory-for-designs	.38	.50	.51
Knox-cubes	.02	.36	.64
learning	.08	.38	.54
incidental-learning	–.15	–.08	.86

poorer. The third component consists primarily of the memory and learning tests.

Although these findings are similar to those of the other factor analytic studies in Africa which were discussed in chapter 3, an important proviso must be made here. The present group of 30 children is not homogeneous as regards age, and age differences may be an important source of the variations in test scores (as shown, the first component correlates highly with age). The other studies were usually carried out either with adults or with groups of children of much smaller age ranges, often with a similar level of education. Therefore, a further analysis was carried out to establish whether an equivalent factor structure remains when the variations due to age differences are removed.[12] The resulting component matrix is presented in table 13. Although the loadings of the individual tests on the components have slightly changed, the overall picture remains the same. The correlation of the first component with education is .51, while the second component has a correlation of –.54 with sex, independent of age. No 'g' factor is found, which is as could be expected, because the Raven-matrices is the only test of general reasoning in the battery. It has also been found repeatedly that among non-western populations, this test correlates rather high with education (Anastasi, 1968, p. 247). Quite naturally the test clusters with the educational tests, vocabulary and arithmetic, and the first component presents a general reasoning/verbal/educational dimension. The spatial-perceptual dimension and the memory-learning dimension are self evident. The memory-for-designs test loads high on the latter two components, which is understandable because the test draws upon both design-copying and short-term memory. For an understanding of later findings, it should be noted that arithmetic is also related to the spatial-perceptual dimension.

Summarizing, it may be concluded that the tests measure different aspects of intellectual functioning, that they group themselves as could be expected from the literature, and that they represent the type of ability for which they were selected.

6. Intellectual Abilities in the Aftermath of Malnutrition

In this chapter the findings of our investigation are discussed in the light of other studies. Before going into more detailed aspects, the evidence deriving from the comparison of previously malnourished with non-malnourished children will first be appraised. The mean test scores for the four groups under study are presented in table 14, while the individual test scores can be found in appendix C. A contrast of the three groups of malnourished children with the comparison group reveals that the first groups score significantly lower on the Raven-matrices, block-design, memory-for-designs[11] and incidental-learning. The differences in the vocabulary, Porteus-mazes, Knox-cubes, and learning show a bias in favour of the comparison children but are not significant. On the arithmetic test, the score of the malnourished children is fractionally above the average score of the comparison children.[13]

Possible interaction effects between malnutrition and sex, and between malnutrition and present age, were calculated and tested for statistical significance. In this part of the analysis twofold divisions were used, first into male and female and secondly into those blocks of children above and those below the median age at the time of study. No interaction effects are found for any test.

The chances that the differences between malnourished and comparison children do not result from malnutrition but from other aspects of the home environment are small. The groups are of the same tribe and sex and nearly identical in age and

Table 14 *Means for tests*

	Malnourished children, age on admission: 8-15 months	16-21 months	22-27 months	Comparison group
Group number	1	2	3	4
Raven-matrices	22.8	21.9	21.5	24.1
vocabulary	7.2	8.6	8.7	9.0
arithmetic	8.8	9.7	9.6	9.3
Porteus-mazes	6.4	6.3	6.2	7.0
block-design	16.7	15.7	16.4	21.9
memory-for-designs (errors)	7.1	8.7	4.4	4.7
Knox-cubes	37.5	38.7	40.7	39.6
learning	3.8	4.5	4.8	5.1
incidental-learning	4.0	5.1	4.6	5.9

Table 15 *Analysis of variance: randomized block design (df = 1,57). F-values resulting from comparison of group 4 (comparison children) with groups 1, 2, and 3 (malnourished children)*

Raven-matrices	F = 4.24*
vocabulary	F = 0.78
arithmetic	F = –0.03
Porteus-mazes	F = 2.66
block-design	F = 8.28**
memory-for-designs	T = 48.5* (a)
Knox-cubes	F = 0.18
learning	F = 1.17
incidental-learning	F = 5.94*

(a) Wilcoxon matched-pairs signed-ranks test.

** $p < .01$.

* $p < .05$.

education. They are also similar in the basic measures of their home environment.

Most studies have found that the intellectual abilities of previously malnourished children are affected. There are some studies of children who were admitted for treatment of malnutrition and who were tested one or two years afterwards (Pollitt and Granoff, 1967; Brockman and Ricciuti, 1971). These children were found to perform less well than comparison children on various cognitive tests – evidence of a short-term effect, the permanency of which needs confirmation from studies in older children.

Many follow-up and longitudinal investigations with older children have often exerted less than sufficient control over the other variables that influence mental development. Some investigators have not used comparison groups of non-malnourished children but have compared the performance of formerly malnourished children with the test norms for the general population (Cabak and Najdanvic, 1965; Mönckeberg, 1968), whilst others have not made certain that the comparison groups that were used were similar with regard to social and economic background (Stoch and Smythe, 1967). Others give insufficient evidence of matching procedures (Liang, Hie, Jan, and Giok, 1967; Champakam, Srikantia, and Gopalan, 1968; Werner and Muralidharan, 1970). Several studies have seriously attempted to eliminate the influence of external variables (Botha-Antoun, Babayan, and Harfouche, 1968; Birch, Pineiro, Alcade, Toca, and Cravioto, 1971; Chase and Martin, 1970; Hertzig *et al.*, 1972; Klein, Lester, Yarbrough, and Habicht, 1975; McLaren, Yaktin, Kanawati, Sabbagh, and Kadi, 1973) and will be discussed in more detail in the next sections. All these studies report that a deficit in test performance is associated with malnutrition. Two studies report contrary findings. Ghai, Ratna, Ramachandran, and Neki (1973) found differences in I.Q. between malnourished children and matched controls, differences that were not statistically significant although they were of a magnitude similar to those found in other studies. Evans, Moodie, and Hansen (1971) failed to find differences in I.Q. between formerly malnourished children and their siblings. Nonetheless, the general picture is that malnourished children show impairment. Since none of these investigations studied adults, the possibility remains that the malnourished children can still catch up by one or both of the twin processes of accelerated development or delayed maturation allowing for a longer period of development in the malnourished children. The lack of interaction between malnutrition and present age found in our study does not support this idea, but the suggestion merits closer attention.

If 'catch-up' occurs among the malnourished children, this means that their test scores should improve over the years, more than the normal increase in test scores occurring over the years among non-malnourished children. Thus, in our study, if 'catch-up' occurs after the age of 11 years, there should be a greater increase in test scores with age among the malnourished than among the comparison children. This stronger relation between age and test scores among the index children should conse-

Table 16 *Partial correlations of age with tests (education constant)*

	malnourished groups (pooled results; N = 3 x 20)	comparison group (N = 20)
Raven-matrices	–.14	–.01
vocabulary	.46**	.25
arithmetic	–.17	–.15
Porteus-mazes	–.08	–.10
block-design	–.28	–.10
memory-for-designs	–.11	–.19
Knox-cubes	–.09	.07
learning	–.03	–.17
incidental-learning	–.08	.05

** $p < .01$, one-tailed test.

quently be reflected in a higher correlation between age and test scores among these children. Because education will also influence test performance, partial correlations, independent of education, were calculated (table 16). The partial correlations of age with eight of the nine tests are neither positive nor significant, with a mean of –.12 among the malnourished children and –.08 in the comparison group. The correlation between vocabulary and age is higher among the malnourished children. This could indeed mean that on this test, the malnourished children are reducing the previously existing differences, since at the time of the testing no differences in vocabulary were found between the index and the comparison children. On the other hand, the difference between the correlations may also be due to chance variations. On the whole, this evidence does not support the idea of a diminishing deficit; instead it indicates that, with the exception of the mastery of Luganda, both groups of children have reached their full development as far as age is concerned[14] and that the deficits of the malnourished children are likely to be permanent.

Up to this point, the focus has been on the overall syndrome of protein-energy malnutrition, but as argued earlier, it is necessary to look more closely at the different characteristics of protein-energy malnutrition.

6.1 Age at malnutrition

Animal studies have demonstrated that there is a 'critical period' of development when malnutrition leads to a permanent deficit or distortion. This period coincides with the brain growth spurt of cell multiplication and myelinization and occurs at different ages in different species (Dobbing, 1974). If the idea of a 'critical period' pertains also to man, this leads to the hypothesis that the severity of the effect of malnutrition will be related to age at onset and the degree to which it overlaps the 'critical period'. In this case it is likely that the younger the child when protein-energy malnutrition occurs, the more severe the ultimate effect. One study did find indications of such a 'critical period'. Cravioto and Robles (1965) studied the recovery of two groups of children: six children who were hospitalized before 6 months of age and nine children hospitalized after 15 months of age. All children were studied within less than 240 days of their admission. The younger group during recovery showed no signs of making up for their initial deficit in test performance, whereas the children admitted at a later age did show some indications of making up their deficit. These results suggest that malnutrition in the early months after birth is more damaging than malnutrition, say, after 12 or 18 months of age. Other studies, however, do not bear this out.

Cabak and Najdanvic (1965) found no correlation between age at the time of illness and subsequent I.Q. in children who were at the time of the study between 7 and 14 years of age, but who had suffered from malnutrition between 4 and 24 months of age.

A study was made of three groups of Jamaican children admitted to the hospital for protein-energy malnutrition: before 7 months of age, between 8 and 12 months, and between 13 and 24 months of age. Several years later, when the children were between 5 and 11 years of age, these groups did not differ in test performance (Hertzig *et al.*, 1972) and school performance (Richardson, Birch, and Hertzig, 1973).

In a study of Lebanese children who were between 3 and 5 years of age, a correlation close to zero was observed between the age at previous admission for malnutrition and the present I.Q. (McLaren *et al.*, 1973).

In a South African study, children hospitalized for malnutrition between 10 and 15 months of age were compared with children admitted between 16 and 48 months. When tested between the ages of 9 and 14 years, the group which had suffered earlier in life did considerably better than the group which had been admitted later in life. The authors suggest that the differences in test performance may have been due to considerable differences in the social environment of the two groups of children (Evans *et al.*, 1971).

All malnourished children in the present study had been admitted before the age of 28 months. Comparison of the children admitted before 16 months of age (group 1) with the children admitted at later ages, between 16-21 and 22-27 months of age

Table 17 *Analysis of variance, randomized block design (df = 1,57). F-values resulting from comparison of groups 2 and 3 (late admissions) with group 1 (early admissions)*

Raven-matrices	F = –1.10
vocabulary	F = 2.44
arithmetic	F = 2.33
Porteus-mazes	F = –0.14
block-design	F = –0.10
memory-for-designs	T = 74.5 [(a)]
Knox-cubes	F = 1.96
learning	F = 1.35
incidental-learning	F = 2.53

(a) Wilcoxon matched-pairs signed-ranks test. n.s.

(groups 2 and 3), tests the hypothesis that early malnutrition has a greater effect than later malnutrition, within this period of 27 months. Analysis of variance shows that there are no significant differences on any of the tests (table 17), and that this is also true for the four tests which showed significant differences between the malnourished and comparison children. The group admitted at the youngest age scores slightly higher on Raven-matrices and block-design but slightly lower on memory-for-designs and incidental-learning than the children admitted at later ages.

In the studies discussed above, the children were usually older than 6 months on admission. This is conceivably past the age of greatest vulnerability. Chase and Martin (1970) compared nine children who were admitted with malnutrition before 4 months of age, with ten children who were admitted between the ages of 5 and 12 months. These groups were identical in their social background. At the age of $3\frac{1}{2}$-$4\frac{1}{2}$ years the group which had suffered early was only slightly behind a matched control group of normal children in development. Contrary to what might be expected the group of children admitted late, between 5 and 12 months, scored far below the group which was early admitted and below the comparison group.

Thus there is almost no evidence[15] that malnutrition occurring after 6 months of age, or even after 12-18 months of age, is less damaging than earlier malnutrition. But here a fundamental problem of interpretation presents itself. The age of the child at first treatment is usually taken to be synonymous with the 'age at onset' of malnutrition. This seems justified with regard to the components of 'acute malnutrition'. The oedema, hypoproteinaemia and skin changes usually precipitate the admission, and the period of time that has elapsed between their onset and first treatment will be negligible. The age at first treatment, however, does not necessarily correspond to the onset of the components of 'chronic undernutrition', which antedate the admission by varying periods. Since it appears that 'chronic undernutrition' is the significant factor responsible for retardation (see below), these studies can shed little light on the role that age plays in the effects resulting from malnutrition.

Since, as described in chapter 1, the pattern of malnutrition occurring in Buganda is rather uniform (weight deficit together with frequent infections commences at the time of weaning, usually between 6 and 12 months of age), one thing can be deduced from the present study. Our findings indicate that the child is still vulnerable at this time, though to what extent this vulnerability depends on interference with the brain growth spurt, on the basis of Dobbing's 'critical period' in animals, remains uncertain. Recent insights from biochemistry and physiology indicate that the 'growth spurt' of the human brain may indeed extend over a much longer period than was formerly thought, e.g. up to two years after birth (Dobbing, 1974).

6.2 Components of malnutrition

Several studies have reported a relation between the degree of wasting or 'chronic undernutrition' and test performance. Cabak and Najdanvic (1965) found a correlation between weight deficit on admission and test performance at the age of 7 to 14 years. Brockman and Ricciuti (1971) studied malnourished children some 12 weeks after recovery and report correlations of .40 between test performance and body length and weight. Among undernourished children aged 3-7 years in Guatemala (Klein *et al.*, 1975), height and head circumference correlated negatively with test performance, independent of the correlation between social environment and test scores. Evans *et al.* (1971) did not find a relation between I.Q. and weight for age at discharge after recovery. (However, this weight reflects the severity of 'chronic undernutrition' less adequately than, for example, the lowest weight during recovery.) As previously discussed, Chase and Martin (1970) found that children who had been admitted between 5 and 12 months of age showed much greater retardation than children who had been admitted before 4 months of age. The authors attribute this to the longer duration of 'chronic undernutrition' in the older children, assuming that the malnutrition commenced shortly after birth. These findings point to a relation between 'chronic undernutrition' and later intellectual abilities. They do not exclude the possibility of the 'acute episode' also having an effect.

In the present study the different effects resulting from the variation in type and severity of malnutrition were analysed within the groups of malnourished children. The severity of 'chronic undernutrition' during the period of admission, and the severity of 'acute malnutrition' on admission, were assessed as described in chapter 4. 'Acute malnutrition' shows no consistent correlations with the tests (table 18). Five of the nine correlations do not exceed (±) .06, while four of the correlations are positive and five are negative. The correlations of 'chronic undernutrition' with the tests are consistently negative; that is the children do less well on the tests the greater the degree of 'chronic undernutrition' in early childhood. For five of the tests these correlations are significant; and although not significant for vocabulary, Porteus-mazes, and learning, they are still negative and larger than .15. Incidental-learning is the one test that fails to show a correlation with 'chronic undernutrition', which is rather surprising since there were significant differences

Table 18 *Correlations of two independent dimensions of malnutrition, 'acute malnutrition' and 'chronic undernutrition', with tests (results of malnourished groups pooled; N = 3 x 20)*

	'Acute malnutrition'	'Chronic undernutrition'
Raven-matrices	.02	–.40**
vocabulary	–.12	–.17
arithmetic	–.05	–.44**
Porteus-mazes	–.06	–.18
block-design	–.02	–.34**
memory-for-designs	–.02	–.33**
Knox-cubes	.17	–.27*
learning	.13	–.21
incidental-learning	.13	–.03

** $p < .01$, one-tailed test.
* $p < .05$, one-tailed test.

between the malnourished and the comparison children on this test. This discrepancy will be discussed later. The fact that 'chronic undernutrition' shows significant negative correlations with test performance later in life indicates that this is the responsible factor and not 'acute malnutrition', which shows no evidence of having an impairing effect.

These results also have a bearing on the interpretation of the studies where siblings were used as comparisons for malnourished children. Since siblings share the same environment, they have presumably experienced similar nutritional circumstances. Although they may have escaped an episode of 'acute malnutrition', the siblings may have suffered similar degrees of less obvious 'chronic undernutrition'. If this is indeed the case we should expect no differences in test performance to occur between them. Four studies have used siblings as comparisons. The differences between siblings reported in two studies (Birch *et al.*, 1971; Hertzig *et al.*, 1972) are difficult to interpret because neither study reports the heights or weights of the children. This makes it impossible to assess the degree to which the siblings may have differed in degree of 'chronic undernutrition'. The siblings in the second study did not, however, differ in school performance (Richardson *et al.*, 1973). The results of one study (Evans *et al.*, 1971) confirm the above argument. Children between 8 and 15 years of age, who had been admitted for protein-energy malnutrition between the ages of 10 and 48 months, did not differ from siblings in somatic growth, nor did they differ in performance on the South African version of the W.I.S.C.. In contrast, McLaren *et al.* (1973) reported no differences in somatic development between children previously admitted to the hospital and siblings, but test performance favoured the latter. These children were then between 3 and 5 years old, and the malnourished children had been admitted to the hospital between 3 and 16 months of age. Perhaps this apparent contradiction arises from the fact that at the time of the study, these children were much younger than the children studied by ourselves and by Evans *et al.* (1971).

6.3 The nature of the intellectual impairment

Some South American studies have emphasized that intersensory integration and language abilities are affected (Cravioto *et al.*, 1966; Cravioto and DeLicardie, 1970; 1972) but these studies do not present findings regarding other abilities. Champakam *et al.* (1968) have, on the contrary, reported that malnourished children showed less impairment on verbal and memory tests than on perceptual tests and tests for abstract reasoning. Unfortunately these authors present only raw scores with no further statistical analysis.

Most studies point to a general impairment of abilities. The verbal and performance subscales of the Wechsler intelligence scales have usually demonstrated similar results (Birch *et al.*, 1971; Evans *et al.*, 1971; Hertzig *et al.*, 1972; Stoch and

Smythe, 1967; Ghai *et al.*, 1973). The Yale Development Scale consists of five subtests assessing five areas of development: gross motor, fine motor, adaptive, language, and personal-social development. The differences in development quotient between malnourished and comparison children reported by Chase and Martin (1970) were nearly identical for all subscales. Botha-Antoun *et al.* (1968) and McLaren *et al.* (1973), using the Stanford-Binet, have reported similar results for parts of the test.

Among undernourished children aged 3-7 years in Guatemala, height and head circumference correlated negatively with test performance, independent of the correlation between social environment and test scores (Klein *et al.*, 1975). The multiple correlation of height and head circumference was highest with tests of perception, intermediate with tests of memory, and lowest with tests of language ability. Our results are remarkably similar to these last findings, although their interpretation presents some difficulties.

Each of the nine tests can be examined in two distinct ways: on the differences between the index and the comparison children, and on the correlation with 'chronic undernutrition' within the three malnourished groups. The two sets of data are usually consistent and show a comparable magnitude of effect for the tests with the exception of arithmetic, Knox-cubes, and incidental-learning. Although arithmetic correlates negatively with 'chronic undernutrition', the test produces no differences whatsoever between the malnourished and the comparison children. This may well result from the educational matching of the four groups. The competence of a child in arithmetic is probably strongly related to the level reached in school. Thus the matching on educational level may have been tantamount to matching on arithmetic competence, without eliminating any negative correlation between arithmetic test score and 'chronic undernutrition' among the malnourished children. The arithmetic test has elements in common with tests of general reasoning and spatial abilities. This has been shown in chapter 5, and is also evident from the high correlations of the test with Raven-matrices and block-design (.65 and .66 among the malnourished children; .38 and .27 among the comparison children). Since in these two abilities the malnourished children are less competent than the comparison children, the malnourished children must have obtained their identical arithmetic scores by another means. This inequality could be compensated for by better concentration, so that they are less easily distracted and they pay less attention to irrelevant information. That these children do indeed pay less attention to irrelevant information is strongly suggested by their lower scores on incidental-learning. Interpreted in this way, the difference between malnourished and comparison children on incidental-learning becomes an artefact of the matching (not necessarily a compensatory mechanism general to malnourished children). This also explains why incidental-learning shows no correlation with 'chronic undernutrition'. The inconsistency in the Knox-cubes results probably arises in a similar way as a consequence of the matching. One inference to be drawn from this argument is that here the nature of the impairment is more accurately reflected by the correlations with 'chronic undernutrition' than by the differences between malnourished and comparison children.

The malnourished children show no overall indications of organic brain damage such as are present in acute- and chronic-brain-disordered patients. They score a mean of 6.7 errors on the memory-for-designs test, which falls considerably below the critical level of 11.5, above which brain damage is suspected according to the U.S. norms. The test, however, shows a high negative correlation with 'chronic undernutrition' together with block-design, Raven-matrices, and arithmetic, indicating that general reasoning and spatial-perceptual abilities are most severely affected. The much lower correlation of the third spatial-perceptual test, Porteus-mazes, with 'chronic undernutrition' is probably a result of using a shortened and less reliable version of this test. Short-term memory (Knox-cubes) and rote learning (learning test) are less severely influenced, while language ability (Luganda vocabulary) appears to be influenced least, if at all.

6.4 Summary

Like many other studies, the present one finds signs of impairment of intellectual abilities in malnourished children and, with the possible exception of one test, finds no signs of 'catch-up' occurring after the age of 11 years. The impairment is found to be independent of the age at which children had been admitted to the hospital, something that was also found in other investigations. The present study further shows that the acute episode, as such, does not contribute to the impairment. Instead it is the degree of 'chronic undernutrition', as distinguished from 'acute malnutrition', that is related to later intellectual abilities – a finding which derives support from the results of other investigations. The results furthermore point to a general impairment of intellectual abilities, with reasoning and spatial abilities most affected, memory and rote learning intermediately affected, and language ability least, if at all, affected.

7. Motor Ability

Studies with malnourished animals have found that the motor function of these animals was affected. Beagle pups, born of normally nourished mothers, who were given protein-deficient diets at weaning showed fine head tremors and a stiff-legged, unsteady gait. These signs of abnormality receded after some months but rarely disappeared. When pups born of malnourished mothers were weaned to low-protein diets, the changes in behaviour were more dramatic: the gait was more severely affected, the tremors were worse, and the animals tired quickly and repeatedly passed into convulsions. After three months this condition improved rapidly, but the recovery was not complete, '... the gait improves, but the legs remain somewhat stiff and wide based ...' (Stewart and Platt, 1968, p. 176.) No such behavioural changes, however, were observed in successive generations of malnourished rats where only occasional tremors and a prolonged sluggish period were observed (Stewart, 1972).

Some studies with malnourished, and previously malnourished, children have also found indications of motor impairment. Cravioto and Robles (1965) reported retardation in motor development, as measured by the Gesell scale, among children malnourished before the age of six months some 200 days later. Normal and malnourished children have also been reported to differ in performance on the visual-motor items of the Stanford-Binet test, when they were between 3 and 5 years of age (McLaren *et al.*, 1973; Werner and Muralidharan, 1970). The Yale Development Scale that was used in the study by Chase and Martin (1970) assesses (apart from adaptive, language, and personal-social development) gross and fine motor abilities. The malnourished children admitted between 5 and 12 months of age showed themselves, at the ages of 3½-4½ years, as much behind in these two aspects of motor development as in cognitive development. Most of these studies were not interested so much in motor development itself as in motor ability as an indicator of development at this early age. Studies of older children have usually concentrated on cognitive abilities and no longer paid attention to motor ability. The assessment of motor function, however, provides an important supplement to the evidence obtained from other tests.

To our knowledge, no studies exist of general motor ability in African teen-age children. The few available studies have been limited to newly born children and infants (see Warren, 1972) or to specific aspects of motor ability among adults such as manual dexterity (De Wet, 1967) or reaction time (Athayde, 1934). Apart from the tests discussed in the previous chapters, all the children in our study were also given the Lincoln-Oseretsky motor development scale, a test covering a wide range of motor abilities during a one-hour individual examination. The test consists of 36 items involving motor skills such as finger dexterity, eye-hand co-ordination, and gross activity of the hands, arms, legs, and trunk. Both unilateral and bilateral tasks are included. The test goes back to an effort by the Russian, N. Oseretsky, to develop a motor equivalent to the Binet test. The initial test had 85 items and was organized by age levels from 4 to 16 years, but the test has since undergone various translations and adaptations. The Lincoln-Oseretsky, one of the last versions, was developed by Sloan (1955), who tested 649 children between the ages 6 and 14 years in the U.S.A.. Those items from the original scale were selected that '(a) could be administered to subjects of both sexes from the ages of six to fourteen years, (b) permitted reliable scoring, (c) minimized cultural bias, (d) involved no danger of injury to the subject, (e) did not require elaborate test materials, (f) had a significant positive correlation with age.' (Sloan, 1955, p. 5.) This led to the exclusion of 49 of the original 85 items, leaving the present version with 36 items that has separate scoring systems for boys and girls. The split-half reliability coefficients that are presented for each age level are usually above .80, often larger than .90, with a median of .86. The reliability coefficients for all boys and all girls of different ages taken together are .96 and .97 respectively. Sloan summarizes his presentation of the scale by concluding that '(a) the test items sample a fairly comprehensive area of motor ability; (b) the test correlates well with age and is capable of discriminating between children of different ages; (c) the items seem to be homogeneous and are saturated in a general factor of maturation and probably other common factors; (d) the test correlates low, but positively, with other tests of motor ability.' (1955, p. 14.)

The original (longer) scale had been designed by Oseretsky to assess six components of motor function, i.e. balance, manual co-ordination, balance while in movement, speed of movements, simultaneous movements with more than one extremity, and absence of superfluous side movements (Vandenberg, 1964). As regards the individual items it is not always clear which of the six components they belong to. Moreover, studies have not succeeded in confirming the existence of the six corresponding subscales within the larger scale. The test also appears to be less sensitive than expected in identifying brain-damaged children, but rather gives an assessment of the general level of motor development (Schilling, 1970; Neuhäuser, 1975). The shorter version of the scale used here, the Lincoln-Oseretsky, has also been the subject of some factor analytic studies which have not, however, yielded convincing results. Findings presented by Vandenberg (1964) suggest the possible existence of a control precision factor, a neurological signs factor, two balance factors, and a co-ordination factor besides some others which defy identification.

7.1 The Lincoln-Oseretsky used with Baganda children

In the present investigation the test was given in its standard form, without any alterations, to all 80 children in the four groups in the study and to the 10 extra children (group 5), previously not malnourished.[16] As with the other tests, the first analysis of the scale was carried out on the basis of the results of the 30 children in groups 4 and 5. The average score for the full scale (36 items) are presented by age level in figure 2. Although the scores of the Baganda children fall below the U.S. standards by some 10-15 points, the age curves appear to be similar. (Standards for U.S. children older than 14 years are not available.) As with the U.S. children, the test is sensitive to age differences among the Baganda children.

Because all the Baganda children were older than 11 years of age, the first items in the scale were passed by all or nearly all of them. Item-total correlations were not computed for the 10 items that were passed by 95% or more of the children in groups 4 and 5; any correlations computed for these items would have had little meaning. Of the 26 items for which item-total correlations (Kendall Tau B) were computed, 3 had correlations lower than .15 and were omitted from the test.[17] The reliability estimate of the remaining test was independently

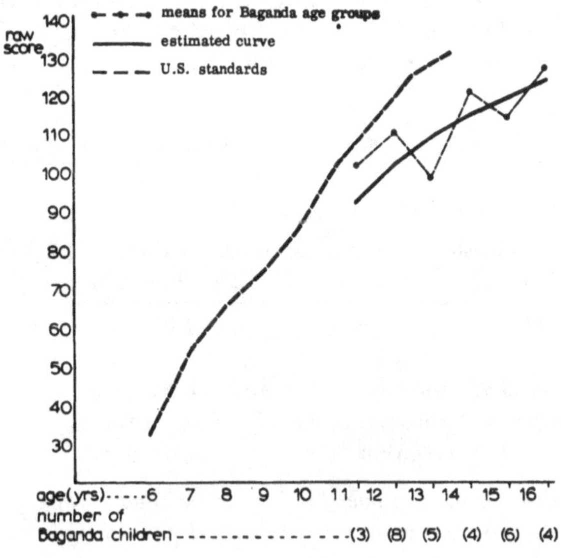

Figure 2 Lincoln-Oseretsky motor development scale: mean scores for Baganda children and U.S. standards.

computed over the 60 malnourished children. The split-half reliability estimate was .80, which is below, but not far below, that reported for the total group of U.S. children of all ages using the 36-item scale.

7.2 The motor function of previously malnourished children

The results of the test for the four groups under study are presented in table 19A. The analysis is similar to that carried out for the other tests. Analysis of variance shows the comparison group to be significantly different from the previously malnourished children. There are, however, no significant differences between the children admitted to the hospital before the age of 15 months and children admitted at later ages (table 19B). Among the 60 malnourished children motor development correlates negatively and significantly with the degree of 'chronic undernutrition' as measured at the time of admission (table 19C). These results are similar to those in the previous chapter. Just as intellectual abilities are affected among previously malnourished children, so also is motor ability.

Table 19 *Results for Lincoln-Oseretsky motor development scale*

A. Means, raw scores:

Malnourished children, age on admission:			Comparison group
8-15 months	16-21 months	22-27 months	
95.3	93.9	97.9	103.8

B. Analysis of variance, randomized block design:
group 4 v. groups 1, 2, 3; $F = 6.69; p < .05$;
groups 2, 3 v. group 1; $F = 0.04$; n.s.

C. Pooled correlation over the 3 malnourished groups (1, 2, 3) of Lincoln-Oseretsky with degree of 'chronic undernutrition' at admission:
$r = -.25$; $p < .05$; one-tailed test.

Further analysis of the individual items may produce insights as to which type of motor ability is most affected. From this analysis, items with a low discriminatory power (that is items that were successfully passed by 90% or more of the children in the index and comparison groups) were excluded, which left 21 items. For these 21 items, the difference between the proportion of comparison children and the proportion of index children passing that item is presented in table 20. The items are listed in the order of the magnitude of this difference with a brief description of each item. Closer inspection of the individual items suggests that they can be distinguished in four types of activity: balancing, jumping, fine movements involving only one hand (FM1), and fine movements involving the independent activity of both hands simultaneously (FM2). The ranking in table 20 indicates that the difference between the malnourished and the comparison children is largest with respect to these latter tasks. Of the six items that show a difference larger than .10, five consist of such tasks requiring the use of both hands. Only one item which involves both hands shows a difference of less than .10. A Mann-Whitney U test confirms that this type of motor ability is most strongly affected ($p < .01$). This finding can not be explained by differences in item difficulty or discriminatory power, since these were not different for these fine movements, when compared with the rest of the items. (It is interesting to note that four of these five items were part of the 'control precision' and the 'neurological signs' factors suggested by Vandenberg (1964), while all five, of course, call to mind Oseretsky's fifth component, that is simultaneous movements with more than one extremity.)

In an attempt to further verify this finding, the scores on the FM1 and FM2 scales were computed for the previously malnourished children and the correlations of these scales with the degree of 'chronic undernutrition' on admission were computed. In the previous chapter it was shown that this, in all probability, is the significant component responsible for intellectual retardation. The correlations were calculated separately for each of the index groups and subsequently pooled. Although the magnitude of both correlations falls below that required for statistical significance, the correlation of 'chronic

Table 20 *Lincoln-Oseretsky: difference between comparison group (c) and malnourished groups (m) in the proportion (p) of children passing individual items* (where items are scored other than just pass or fail, the proportion is calculated as the obtained score divided by the maximum possible score)

Item number and description	Type of motor activity (*)	$p_c - p_m$
(16) describing circles in the air with both index fingers simultaneously	FM2	.25
(31) tapping alternately with feet and describing circles in the air with both index fingers simultaneously	FM2	.20
(34) balancing on tiptoe of one leg	B	.19
(10) closing and opening hands alternately and simultaneously	FM2	.15
(20) putting matchsticks in one box with two hands simultaneously	FM2	.12
(18) putting coins and matchsticks in two boxes with two hands simultaneously	FM2	.11
(26) putting coins in box with one hand	FM1	.09
(27) tracing mazes with pencil	FM1	.09
(25) cutting a circle with scissors	FM1	.08
(30) jumping and touching heels with both hands	J	.08
(35) opening and closing hands simultaneously	FM2	.07
(19) jumping, making an about turn, landing on tiptoes and holding balance	J + B	.07
(21) winding thread while walking	FM1	.07
(13) rolling piece of paper into a ball	FM1	.06
(23) putting matchsticks on piles with one hand	FM1	.06
(14) winding thread	FM1	.05
(24) drawing lines between other lines	FM1	.05
(33) jumping and clapping hands	J	.05
(17) tapping dots with pencil	FM1	.02

Item number and description	Type of motor activity	$p_c - p_m$
(32) stand on one foot with eyes closed	B	.02
(36) balancing a rod vertically on index finger	FM1	.01

(*) FM2 = fine movements involving two hands simultaneously
FM1 = fine movements involving one hand
B = balancing
J = jumping

undernutrition' with the FM2 scale is larger (–.22) than the correlation with the FM1 scale, which is nearly nil (–.03). Thus the idea remains that the malnourished children are particularly affected in tasks requiring simultaneous, but independent, activity of both hands, which demands lateral co-ordination and discrimination.

8. Aspects of Daily Behaviour

The existing knowledge about the place that mentally retarded children and adults occupy in non-western societies is meagre. What little is known has been laboriously brought together by Edgerton (1970), whom we will briefly follow. He examines some of the conventional assumptions about the retarded in these societies against the information that is available about several African, Asian, and North American Indian societies. The first of these assumptions, that profoundly retarded persons in primitive societies are killed, knows its antonym in the equally widespread idea that in these societies even the most severely retarded are well treated.[18] That the retarded would go unnoticed in non-western societies rests upon the notion that these societies place very few demands upon their members, which is a naïve view. The assumption that in non-western societies the retarded are not stigmatized appears to be equally unjustified: in fact, they often seem to be the victims of discrimination and are often regarded as problems. Some of the information that Edgerton relies on, concerns African tribes. The Pokot of Kenya and the Hehe of Tanzania, for example, recognize mild degrees of stupidity, and they even have a word for such persons. There is even the suggestion that the attitudes towards the mildly retarded are related to ecological variation, to the demands that are imposed by the physical environment. From his own observations in East Africa, Edgerton relates that:

> In both the pastoral and the farming zones, intelligence, cleverness and verbal skill were prized, yet the pastoralists who lived in the more stressful environment were substantially more critical of stupidity than were the farmers. In addition, although I was able to attempt no systematic epidemiological research, I observed far more apparent ... mental retardates in farming areas than I saw in the pastoral areas ... a good many pastoralists sent their retarded children to relatives ... among the nearby mountain-dwelling farmers. (1970, p. 541.)

Some African tribes have developed a folklore about the retarded and assign a special place to them. In East Africa, the clans under whose responsibility the retarded often come, may arrange for someone, often a child, to watch over them to prevent accidents. Here we leave Edgerton's review.

That traditional societies place very few demands upon their members is a notion based upon a naïve view of these societies, as has already been said. A member of an African tribe must, to mention only a few things, be familiar with the genealogy of the people around him for generations back – and if he happens to live in a pastoral society, the genealogy of the cattle belonging to the tribe as well. He has to master the rules of land use and land ownership, which may be of an extreme intricacy and delicacy. Furthermore, there are a multitude of social and economic obligations often partially fulfilled, that may go back for generations with which he must be conversant. The Baganda, for instance, highly value 'amagezi' or intelligence. The word 'amagezi' in Luganda has connotations of understanding (kutegeera) and measuring, evaluating (okugera) (Wober, 1974, p. 264). The Baganda also distinguish 'obusiru' or foolishness which 'is recognised to be of two types, congenital and acquired, and is used for people whose behaviour appears to be that of someone considerably younger than he actually is.' (Orley, 1970, p. 6.)

Traditional Kiganda society had an official training and promotion ladder for boys, and cleverness was rewarded as described in an early ethnographic account:

> When about ten, they [boys] were expected to perform light duties such as carrying their relative's beer and mat,

> or going messages for him. If the relative saw that the boy was bright and quick he would possibly get him into the household of some chief; there the boy, if he was attentive, might soon make his way and become a trusted servant, and be sent upon important business. He might even become a page to the King, and in this position, if he gained favour by his alertness, promotion would be certain. (Roscoe, 1911, pp. 75-6.)

Brightness could take a boy or a man far in life, and status mobility among the Baganda is not a recent phenomenon, as the following account shows:

> Since well before the establishment of British administration, a process of progressive political centralization had increasingly opened positions of power and wealth to men of talent. Rising to a position of influence through loyal and able service to a lord was both culturally approved and empirically possible, and in the course of the nineteenth century was becoming ever easier and more acceptable. (Fallers, 1964, p. 159.)

It is not surprising that the introduction of formal education was positively received among the Baganda. On the one hand it interfered with the traditional system of social mobility, but on the other it enforced mobility by providing another means of achieving élite status. Mobility was not determined exclusively by merit; there were greater possibilities open to children of chiefs and the nobility than to children of common farmers. Yet these avenues to prosperity and respect were open to all (Fallers, 1964, pp. 161-2).

The above does not imply that previously malnourished children are necessarily perceived as (mildly) retarded in Kiganda society. In fact, from informal observations, there were no indications that these children were perceptibly different from their peers. Nevertheless, information about the day-to-day behaviour of these children in their homes was collected by means of interviews with the parents. Since we did not in any way wish to antagonize the parents we refrained from enquiring how bright the children were. After all, that was what *we* had come to assess, and such questions might easily have been interpreted as negative judgements and have led to misunderstandings. Instead we concentrated on other aspects of the children's behaviour, including the chores they performed at home. Two questionnaires were verbally presented, in Luganda, to the parent who was at home during the psychological examination of the child. This was usually the mother.

8.1 Household jobs

The initial list consisted of 12 tasks that boys and girls may perform in the Kiganda home. The parents had to reply whether the child performed a job either with a simple yes or no; or with a never, sometimes, or often, whichever was applicable. Analysis of the individual items was carried out over the 30 children in groups 4 and 5 which had not been admitted for malnutrition during early childhood. The response categories of the questions with more than two possible answers were dichotomized so that the division fell nearest to 50%. For some items, this still meant that more than 90% of the responses fell in one category. These items were omitted as were the questions which did not apply to more than only a few children. Guttman scaling finally left eight items which compose the household jobs scale (table 21). This scale has a coefficient of reproducibility of .75 as independently calculated over the 60 previously malnourished children, indicating that it is largely unidimensional. For each task performed one point was added to the score, so that theoretically the total could fall between 0 and 8; and in fact among the 30 children in groups 4 and 5, the lowest score was 0 and the highest score 8.

The average number of jobs performed by the malnourished children is 3.9, that performed by the comparison children is 3.1.[19] Analysis of variance, randomized block design, shows that this difference is not significant (F= –2.20). The hint that previously malnourished children do more jobs is not confirmed by further analysis among the index children. The (pooled) correlation of 'chronic undernutrition' with the jobs performed is only –.01. Thus the impairment resulting from 'chronic undernu-

Table 21 *Household jobs in final scale*

- to wash parent's clothes
- to clean the house
- to wash the plates
- to fetch water
- to fetch firewood
- responsibility for a part of the garden
- to go shopping
- to take care of the house and the younger children, at night, when the adults are away.

trition' does not seem to influence the child's participation in these, admittedly simple, household activities, and in this regard, the previously malnourished children appear to function quite normally.

8.2 Behaviour ratings

After pilot testing, 17 questions were left that were concerned with the impression that other people have of the children. These questions had been selected to cover three aspects of the children's behaviour: activity, independence, and friendships. Some questions were opposites of each other, others were nearly identical, while still others covered more or less the same ground. The questionnaire was purposely designed in this way to provide checks on the meaning of the individual questions, through the correlations with other questions. Two questions were omitted because they gave rise to misunderstandings. The first analysis of the remaining questions was, again, carried out with the help of the data obtained from the 30 children in groups 4 and 5. The response categories were dichotomized so that the division fell nearest to 50%. Those questions that still had more than 90% responses in one category were omitted. One item that failed to show a significant correlation with any of the remaining questions was also omitted. This left 12 questions which were arbitrarily subdivided although note was taken of their correlations. They were combined into one group of three questions and four groups of two questions, with one question left on its own. This provides information about six aspects of the children's behaviour that are judged by the parents, and which will be called:

Resting	(1 question) –	Does he (she) often rest during the day;
Slowness	(2 questions) –	Is he slow; Is he quick with jobs;
Activity	(2 questions) –	Does he tire easily; Is he always busy;
Shyness	(2 questions) –	Is he spontaneous; Is he shy;
Obedience	(2 questions) –	Is he obedient; Is he submissive;
Friendships	(3 questions) –	Does he want to be by himself; Does he have few friends; Does he make friends easily.

In an attempt to validate these 'scales' as much as possible, mutual correlations and the correlations with 'household jobs', sex, and age were computed (table 22). These correlations are in accord with the meaning of these scales at face value. Children that are judged to be slow are also judged as not active and as shy, while they also tend to rest more. Active children have more friends. The children that are looked upon as active and obedient are the ones that do most household chores. That girls are more obedient than boys and have fewer friends at this age is characteristic not only of Baganda girls. That they are also judged to be less active than boys is intriguing. Older children are also judged as less active and have fewer friendships. For the latter there is no immediate explanation, but it may indicate that with age, Baganda children become more selective in their social relations. Some parents, in fact, told us that they encouraged their children not to befriend certain children.

For each of these aspects the percentage of children who attained the maximum score was computed[19] in order to test possi-

Table 22 *Correlations (Kendall Tau B) between behaviour ratings, household jobs, sex, and age (Groups 4 and 5; N = 30)*

	resting	slowness	activity	shyness	obedience	household jobs	sex	age
resting	–					.03	.05	.08
slowness	.27*	–				.11	.21	–.03
activity	–.24	–.38**	–			.26*	–.27*	–.30*
shyness	–.01	.23	–.14	–		–.04	–.06	–.06
obedience	–.13	.06	.14	.14	–	.41**	.25	–.08
friendships	–.17	–.13	.26*	.09	.00	–.02	–.47**	–.29*

** $p < .01$.
* $p < .05$.

ble differences for statistical significance. Table 23 presents the results for the comparison children and for all the malnourished children grouped together. There are (near) significant differences on two aspects. The malnourished children rest more and are also judged to be more obedient. Further analysis among the malnourished children confirms this: the degree of 'chronic undernutrition' at admission correlates significantly not only with resting and obedience, but also with activity and slowness (table 24). There is no relation with the ratings for shyness and friendships. These findings, tentative as they are, nevertheless suggest that the activity of the malnourished children is somewhat affected while they also seem to be more obedient. They appear as somewhat docile, less energetic children, but this does not seem to influence the household chores they perform or their relations with others.

There is one other study which has investigated the behaviour of previously malnourished children. Richardson and others (1972) compared 58 such boys with 58 classmates of the same age. The teachers filled in questionnaires about these children, while a sociometric study was also conducted. The previously malnourished boys fared worse on nearly all the aspects touched

Table 23 *Behaviour ratings: percentage of children attaining maximum score*

	Malnourished children (N = 57)	Comparison children (N = 20)
resting	32	10 (a)
slowness	19	20
activity	54	55
shyness	26	25
obedience	88	65 (b)
friendships	32	20 (c)

Cochran Q test: (a) $Q = 9.55$; $p < .05$.
(b) $Q = 7.13$; $p = .06$.
(c) $Q = 2.34$; n.s.

Table 24 *Correlations (Kendall Tau B) of 'chronic undernutrition' with behaviour ratings (results of malnourished groups pooled; N = 3 x 19 = 57)*

resting	.21*
slowness	.19*
activity	–.21*
shyness	.05
obedience	.19*
friendships	.03

* $p < .05$; two-tailed test.

upon in the teacher questionnaire: behaviour related to class work, social relationships, and conduct problems. These children were judged to have poorer memories and to be more easily distracted, less forthcoming, and less co-operative. Their teachers also regarded them as quieter and more withdrawn and reported more behavioural problems. These boys also received less sociometric choices than the comparison boys. These differences are more wide-ranging and more striking than those found in our study. Perhaps the deficits resulting from malnutrition in early childhood are a greater handicap in school than at home, although Richardson *et al.*, (1973) report elsewhere that these boys are not behind their siblings in school results.

9. Conclusions and Speculations

Against the background of our own findings we have tried to provide a framework for the existing psychological evidence concerning the relation between malnutrition and intellectual abilities. By now, the first results of several long-term investigations in South America are also appearing in print. The proceedings of a recent symposium on *'Early Malnutrition and Mental Development'* organized by the Swedish Nutrition Foundation (1974) cover some recent findings and thinking in this field. Some papers presented at this symposium have already been mentioned, but others may serve to provide further insights.

A brief recapitulation of certain features of our investigation may serve to put the findings in a proper perspective. The children studied were relatively mature, 14 years on average; they all belonged to the same tribe and, in this respect, constituted a homogeneous group. We were also able to match the different groups successfully in terms of their socio-economic background. The tests that were used were carefully adapted or constructed, analysed in detail and cover a wide range of abilities. All the children had attended school for some time (four years on average), so that they were not unfamiliar with test situations. Moreover, the testing was always carried out by the same person, that is, either the psychologist or the paediatrician and never left to assistants.[20]

The investigation was carried out by relatively modest means and the staff involved was purposely kept to a minimum. This, on the other hand, made 'blind' testing impossible because we had personally to direct the tracing and selection of children. Nevertheless 'tester bias' does not offer an explanation for the findings. First, we had ample experience in examining children and observed strict rules for each test. Secondly, if bias has occurred, it should have done so in the opposite direction because, if anything, we favoured the view that malnutrition had *no* permanent effects. The decisive refutation of possible 'tester bias' is that this author never examined the medical files of the malnourished children beforehand, and was therefore completely unaware of the seriousness of the children's condition at previous admission. This medical information was copied from the files and analysed only long after the completion of the examinations. Thus the degrees of 'chronic undernutrition' and 'acute malnutrition' suffered many years previously were not known during the examination.

In summary, our most important findings are listed below.

(a) Previously malnourished children show signs of (permanent) impairment when compared, at the ages of 11-17 years, with children of the same sex, age, and education coming from a comparable social environment.

(b) This impairment shows a strong relation with an index, composed of weighted medical indicators, measuring the degree of 'chronic undernutrition' at admission.

(c) No such relation exists with a similar index assessing the degree of 'acute malnutrition' or metabolic imbalance on admission.

(d) The impairment is independent of the age at which the children were admitted to the hospital, between 8 and 27 months.

(e) There is a general impairment of intellectual abilities, with reasoning and spatial abilities most affected, memory and rote learning intermediately affected, and language ability least, if at all, affected.

Findings from other research, as far as they pertain to these central questions, by and large confirm the deleterious influence of 'chronic undernutrition'. The generalization of this finding in respect of children who are not admitted to the hospital for severe malnutrition requires consideration. 'Chronic undernutrition', however, occurs over a period of time prior to the admission. As we have found, the fact that a child ultimately suffers or does not suffer from an 'acute' condition has no effect on his later intellectual abilities. Consequently, children who are 'chronically undernourished', but who never fall 'acutely' ill, must experience similar negative consequences. Research among such children, who have never been subject to acute malnutrition, has confirmed that there is a positive correlation between somatic growth and various aspects of intellectual performance (Klein, Yarbrough, Lasky, and Habicht, 1974).

Waterlow and Rutishauser (1974) plead for a distinction between two types of malnutrition, 'stunting' and 'wasting'. Growth failure or 'stunting' of height, with corresponding lower weight, results from undernutrition over time. On the other hand, 'wasting' of body weight, according to these authors, is an acute condition arising over a short period. In practice, most malnourished children show a combination of these two, so that according to this view, a low weight reflects the combined effects of the 'chronic' and the 'acute' condition. Other authors do not draw such a sharp distinction but regard 'acute malnutrition' as a metabolic imbalance superimposed on long-term growth failure (Rao, 1974). In that case a low weight may result largely from the chronic undernutrition which the child has experienced.

Although the heights of the children in our study had not been recorded at admission, our findings seem to agree with this latter view more than the former. An analysis of the medical indicators recorded at admission showed little relation between low weight and metabolic imbalance. Instead low weight was related to the absence of (oedematous) weight loss after admission and low haemoglobin level. Whatever way may be the best to assess the degree of 'chronic undernutrition', the basic suggestion of Waterlow and Rutishauser that different types of malnutrition should be distinguished remains. In fact the evidence, from this and other studies, that 'chronic undernutrition' and not 'acute malnutrition' damages intellectual abilities already carries the argument a step further.

9.1 Confounding variables

However strong the case for establishing a relation between 'chronic undernutrition' in early childhood and later intellectual abilities, there is always the possibility of alternative explanations. Because of the limitations and imperfections of research in this field, other confounding variables may have contributed to both the lower nutritional status and the lower intellectual abilities. We will look at the four alternative influences which are most often suggested.

(a) *Low birth weight.* This argument runs as follows. The intellectual abilities of children with low birth weights are negatively affected, and these children also suffer more easily from malnutrition. The lower intellectual abilities of malnourished children must really be attributed to the earlier influences that also resulted in the lower birth weights. However, some studies that have actually taken birth weight into account (Chase and Martin, 1970; DeLicardie and Cravioto, 1974) still find impairment to occur with malnutrition. Moreover the hypothesis that children with low birth weights are permanently affected appears due for reconsideration. A case in point is that of the boys who were born during and shortly after the Dutch famine in World War II, when birth weights dropped considerably, who showed no signs of reduced intellectual performance around the age of 18 years (Stein, Susser, Saenger, and Marolla, 1972).

(b) The *genetic argument* is similar to the previous one, except that it suggests some kind of genetically determined 'vitality' and that children with less of it not only have lower intellectual capacities but also more easily fall prey to malnutrition. This argument holds that the less intelligent children suffer more from malnutrition. Apart from the fact that there is little positive evidence for such a phenomenon, some studies that have attempted to take the intellectual abilities of the parents into account (McLaren *et al.*, 1973; Botha-Antoun *et al.*, 1968) still reveal defects accompanying the malnutrition. Attempts to identify future patients have generally also been unsuccessful, which would seem unlikely if these children were really less endowed. More pertinent answers must be provided by longitudinal studies in which children have been observed from birth onwards, although the lack of valid measuring instruments at this early age will remain a serious handicap. There are also indications (see below) that children who are malnourished before 4-6 months of age, are not or are less affected, and this is difficult to reconcile with a genetic explanation.

(c) *Social environment.* This is an explanation that has been suggested time and again. Consequently, it is also one that most researchers give due consideration, yet they still report that impairment accompanies malnutrition. Some critics maintain that all these attempts to control for the social environment must be insufficient because there must be certain characteristics of the social environment which have led to the occurrence of malnutrition in certain children and not in others. This argument loses much of its strength when the culprit is chronic undernutrition which is often widespread among the population. We have also described how in Uganda a child from a quite ordinary environment not only can fall prey to acute malnutrition, but is also subject to chronic undernutrition. One aspect of the social environment, however, requires closer inspection.

(d) *Maternal care and stimulation.* If neglect by the mother is responsible for malnutrition among young children (a view which we do not share, although it may apply in some instances), this also implies less attention and less stimulation for the young child, and offers an alternative explanation for reduced intellectual abilities. This suggestion received fresh support from the findings of a longitudinal study among 330 Mexican children observed from birth onwards (DeLicardie and Cravioto, 1974). Some 14 children developed acute malnutrition despite the fact that they were regularly examined and the parents were given frequent advice. The family background of this group differed in only one aspect from that of a comparison group: at the age of 6 months these children received less stimulation in their homes. This lack of social, emotional, and cognitive stimulation was also evident at later ages, which tempts one to conclude that insufficient care plays a major role in the occurrence of malnutrition.

There are pitfalls in such an interpretation. This group is surely exceptional in that, despite the help and supervision provided by the research team, the children still became severely malnourished. Perhaps these mothers were unco-operative or did indeed neglect their children. It follows, however, that in those cases where the medical team succeeded in preventing malnutrition from occurring, maternal neglect did not play a decisive role. The generalization of this finding is therefore suspect.

Secondly, stimulation is a two-sided process, an interaction between mother and child, in which the child also plays its role. The possibility exists that lack of stimulation is a result of undernutrition, not the reverse. As a first adaptation to undernutrition, children may reduce their energy output, making them less responsive; consequently, the mother becomes less stimulating. DeLicardie and Cravioto (1974, p. 151) seem to recognize such a possible relation between stimulus deprivation and passive behaviour later in life, but it may equally well apply before the occurrence of acute malnutrition. In fact, one of the major changes observed in a supplementation program among infants was that these children became much more energetic, placing more demands upon the mother, to such an extent that these mothers were hardly able to cope with their vigorous children (Chavez, Martinez, and Yaschine, 1974). This brings us to the point where we may try to speculate on the possible ways in which 'chronic undernutrition' affects intellectual abilities.

9.2 Mode of influence

'Chronic undernutrition' has two components, the degree of faltering and the duration of such faltering. There is little evidence that one of these two is the more important, although some faltering and a duration of some time are both inherent to 'chronic undernutrition'. In retrospect, it is usually not possible to distinguish between the respective contributions of these two components to the final condition of a child. The lack of positive findings among children in western countries who for strictly medical reasons became malnourished suggests that duration is important (Lloyd-Still, Hurwitz, Wolff, and Shwachman, 1974; Valman, 1974). After the age of 5 years these children showed no difference in test performance when compared with their siblings. Although both studies have certain weaknesses they recall similar findings by Chase and Martin (1970), who also observed no effects among children malnourished before the age of 4 months.[21] The idea that children who were malnourished very early in life show no, or little, damage gains some support from animal studies. Monkeys in whom malnutrition was induced after cerebral development was largely accomplished still showed lasting behavioural effects (Zimmermann, Geist, Strobel, and Cleveland, 1974). Riopelle (1974) suggests that the infantile nervous system is remarkably plastic and probably less vulnerable than has been thought. There are, however, other explanations that can be offered for the possible lack of permanent effects of malnutrition during the first months of life. The first is that in very young children malnutrition simply has not lasted long enough to have measurable effects. The other explanation might be that malnutrition impairs intellectual abilities by way of experiential deprivation, which possibly becomes important only after 6 months of age.

This leads to the question whether experiential deprivation plays a major role or whether brain growth is directly affected by lack of nutrients. The two are, of course, not mutually exclusive, but may accompany each other and even reciprocally influence each other.

The evidence from psychological studies that the brain is directly affected by malnutrition is meagre. There are no reliable findings which point to gross organic damage. Our finding that previously malnourished children perform better than chronic brain-disordered patients on a test for organic impairment is very pertinent. The fact that most studies find a rather uniform and general retardation could support this. In this instance, the comparison is with gross brain damage but the possibility remains that the brain is affected in less dramatic ways. Dobbing

(1974) argues that if brain growth is affected by malnutrition, it is not the number of neurons that is reduced, even if this does have functional significance. Neuronal multiplication in the human brain occurs during the second intrauterine trimester, a time when the organism is probably highly protected. Afterwards the 'brain growth spurt' consists of glial cell division and myelinization, and later of dendritic growth and branching and the establishing of synaptic connections. Dobbing (1974) suggests that these last processes are more likely to be affected by malnutrition. Our findings regarding motor ability, that malnutrition interferes most with the skills requiring lateral integration could be interpreted as being in support of this. The minor trend observed in some studies (including the present one) that spatial abilities are most affected could be similarly interpreted. This process of the branching and connecting of neurons seems to continue at least until 2 years of age. If indeed the duration of the malnutrition is of major importance, this suggests that the brain can withstand negative conditions to a considerable extent. All in all, the evidence from psychological studies that the brain is directly affected remains exceedingly small. A definite answer will, however, not be found soon, considering the lack of knowledge of the relation between the brain and its function. There is also the possibility that experiential deprivation in its turn may lead to organic changes, while the remarkable plasticity of the brain and its capacity to adapt to adverse circumstances further complicates matters.

Of course, the Mexican children who became so vigorous under a supplementation regime offer no small evidence of the crucial links between malnutrition, reduced energy, apathy, and lack of stimulation in the undernourished child. The mothers of these children had received supplementary foods during pregnancy and lactation, while the children themselves were weaned to a diet of milk and baby foods. These children were somewhat heavier at birth and superior as regards growth and performance on the Gesell tests, and showed, in particular, more physical activity (recorded by time sampling methods) than the comparison children (Chavez *et al.*, 1974).

This suggests that poor nutrition leads to adaptation, which depresses physical activity, something which has indeed been found among Ugandan children (Rutishauser and Whitehead, 1972). This, in turn, limits the interaction of the child with its environment, eventually resulting in retarded intellectual development. Although it is not possible at this stage to conclude positively that such a causal chain exists, the suggestion by Pollitt (1973) that lethargy of the infant may also play a role in the causation of marasmus points in the same direction.

The platitude that research raises more questions than it answers applies in this case, except that the questions can now be formulated in more detail. We are left with a number of possibilities. The brain may be directly affected, and in that case it is likely that the duration of the malnutrition is of prime importance. Stimulus deprivation probably plays an important role, in which case the duration of the process may be equally important. One would not expect permanent impairment to result from a short period of deprivation. There is, however, also the possibility that deprivation will become important only after the first few months of life. If experiential deprivation is indeed crucial, and we think that it is, the reduced energy expenditure by malnourished children requires more study. The tendency has been to regard these reductions as occurring concurrently with growth failure. The more the growth failure the greater the reduction in energy output, which means that the degree of 'growth failure' will be similar to the degree of deprivation. There is, however, the possibility that the reduction in energy output is the first adaptation to poor nutrition and that it occurs before growth retardation. In that case, all children showing growth retardation would first have experienced a similar degree of energy reduction, and variations will occur only in duration.

It follows that research should pay particular attention to the period before and during the first stages of growth retardation. But if reduced energy and stimulation are indeed responsible, attention should also be given to the possibility of this occurring in the toddler age as well. Among Guatemalan children, however, no improvement resulted from diet supplementation after the age of 5 years (Klein *et al.*, 1974). Yet older children also require study because of some tentative suggestions that malnourished children develop a different life style and are characterized by passive behaviour, as reported by DeLicardie and Cravioto (1974) and found in the present study, or that they are less motivated (Klein *et al.*, 1974).

Viewed in this way malnutrition is no longer a cataclysmic event suddenly crippling an infant for life. Instead malnutrition takes its place among the influences that accumulate and interact over long periods of time, even if, in our view, malnutrition plays a crucial role.

9.3 Intervention

Two important inferences can be drawn. First, since 'chronic undernutrition' has a deleterious influence on intellectual abilities, treatment of 'acute cases' is insufficient to prevent impairment. Preventive measures can be effective only when introduced early in the process. Secondly, not only those children are endangered who eventually fall acutely ill, but also those children suffering from less obvious 'chronic undernutrition'. Estimates of the number of children who show signs of such undernutrition in developing countries vary, but are generally high – in the order of 40% or more (Bengoa, 1973).

Before concluding that there is a need for intervention early in the process, it must be noted that although reduced growth results from adverse nutritional circumstances, it can be regarded as an adaptation of man to the environment in which he is placed. Any attempts at intervention in this particular aspect of the growth and development of children is therefore apt to have wider ramifications, apart from the question whether drastic improvements on a large scale are indeed feasible. Such wider ramifications may, for example, include decreased infant mortality but may also lead to increased demands being placed upon the resources of a country. It is necessary to consider whether countries can meet such demands not only now, but also in the future. Economists take a hard and factual view of such matters, asking whether investments in improving nutrition give a greater economic return than investments in other areas (Savosnick, 1972). Some authors have therefore attempted to assess the benefits in increased human potential that can be expected to result from improved nutrition not only among young children, but also in older children and adults (Barg, 1973; Wilson, 1973). Alan Berg in *The Nutrition Factor* has given a concise and reasoned exposé of this dilemma, concluding that 'not only is malnutrition a consequence of underdevelopment but it is a contributing factor, a drag on the potential from which better nutrition might be provided.' (1973, p. 195.) He strongly advocates a central nutrition policy by governments and pleads for such varying approaches as price policies, seed improvement, the distribution of special children's foods through marketing channels, and particularly food fortification. Each of these approaches has its own limitations, of which we mention the experience with the much-heralded commercial weaning foods such as Faffa in Ethiopia and Incaparina in Guatemala. These foods have by and large failed to reach the most needy part of the population for whom they were initially intended.

The emphasis has for a long time been on the need for increased protein consumption, but recently this approach has been severely criticized. McLaren even speaks of the 'great protein fiasco' since, in his opinion, emphasis has unjustly been placed on protein insufficiency to the neglect of calorie insufficiency, with the result that most of the measures that were taken have been inappropriate. He argues that 'an energy gap rather than a protein gap is the crux of the matter'. (McLaren, 1974, p. 95.) If this is indeed the case, and the changing ideas on the evolution of malnutrition point in a similar direction (Rao, 1974), the problem of malnutrition will have to be attacked on a much wider front instead of concentrating on certain nutrients. Diets as a whole will have to be improved, which makes the case for centralized intervention programmes all the less promising. If efforts are undertaken by central governments or international agencies, it is wise if they emphasize increasing and improving local food resources, whereby families are helped to provide for themselves wherever possible. Such efforts have, of course, been a part of agricultural extension and nutrition education, whenever the aim has been to achieve the best results with the food resources that are locally available. A 'low-profile' approach of this nature is attractive because it keeps interference with the social environment at a relative minimum and because it is least abrupt. On the other hand, it requires greater efforts, while the results will be far from spectacular and slow to appear. Nevertheless, these attempts deserve far more serious attention from social scientists than they have received until now.

Notes

1. This section relies upon data presented in the *Atlas of Uganda* (1967) and Langlands (1974), unless indicated otherwise.
2. *The Mountain People* by Colin Turnbull (1972) presents a horrifying account of famine among the Ik, a tribe of hunters and gatherers in northern Karamoja district who have been displaced from their homelands.
3. The percentages that are actually reported by Dean and Burgess (1962) are all ten times higher but it appears that an error was made in connection with the decimal point. The percentages that are presented here are calculated from the raw figures presented by Burgess (1962 a, b, c, d, e), dividing the total number of observed cases by the number of children older than 8 months and younger than 5 years of age.
4. A detailed discussion of descriptive developmental strategies is presented by K. Warner Schaie (1965). For a general discussion of methodological issues in life-span developmental psychology see Nesselroade and Reese (1973).
5. This erroneous interpretation by the authors must find its cause in the cumbersome and elaborate way in which the results are presented, without further statistical analysis. Children had to compare *identical* and *non-identical* forms, each presented in three different combinations of sense modalities; *visual-haptic*, *visual-kinaesthetic*, and *haptic-kinaesthetic*, six conditions in all. The results for these six conditions are not only presented separately, but are also specified for six age groups: 6, 7, 8, 9, 10, and 11 years. Thus, in all, a comparison of the mean number of errors of the tall and short children is presented for 36 occasions for the rural and the urban group. Among the rural children, the mean number of errors of the short children is larger on 29 occasions, on 4 occasions there is

no difference with that of the taller children, while 3 times the taller children make more errors. Thus, the first part of the authors' conclusion that 'among rural children differences in height are accompanied by differences in intersensory integrative ability' is correct. But the rest of the conclusion that *'this is not the case among upper-class children'* (Cravioto *et al.*, 1966, p. 352) is unwarranted. Among the upper-class children the mean number of errors of the short children is larger on 23 occasions, 5 times there is no difference with that of the taller children, while on 8 occasions the taller children make more errors. Among the upper-class children there is a similar trend for tall children to do better than short children, although this trend appears slightly stronger among the rural children, particularly at younger ages.

6. The authors furthermore fail to take account of the resulting distribution of test scores in the statistical analysis.
7. This chapter is concerned with Africa, south of the Sahara, or black Africa as it is also called. This delimitation is necessary not only because of the cultural differences with the north of the continent, but also because the bulk of the existing psychological literature concerns those inhabitants found south of the Sahara (Marais and Hoorweg, 1971). For reasons of convenience, the general terms Africa and Africans are used in the text.
8. Since MacDonald's work has never been published this information is taken from the presentation by Grant and Schepers (1969).
9. The particulars and the test scores of the children in group 5 are listed in appendix E.
10. The scoring of the memory-for-designs test relies largely upon the judgement of the scorer. The drawings produced by the children have to be rated by comparison with examples presented in the manual. All 15 drawings by each of the 90 children in groups 1-5 were independently rated by two scorers who relied exclusively upon the manual. The total test score of each child was thus computed twice. The correlation between the scores given by the two judges was .90.
11. The memory-for-designs test has a skewed distribution of scores. To allow for this distribution, scores on this test were dichotomized where correlational analysis is used in chapters 5 and 6. An error score of 5 or higher was recoded into 0; when the error score was 4 or lower, it was recoded 1. Furthermore, instead of an analysis of variance as used with the other tests in chapter 6, for this test Wilcoxon's signed ranks test for matched pairs is utilized.
12. The actual calculations were as follows. First, the component

matrix (A), presented in table 12A, was rotated, so that the correlation of age with the second (II) and third (III) component became .00. These two components are thus independent of age.

In the next step, the partial correlations between all nine tests were computed, with age kept constant. From this matrix, the two previously calculated components, II and III, which are independent of age (once they were corrected for removed variance) were subtracted. The diagonal values were also adjusted for the removal of these two components. From the residual matrix, the first principal component (I) was calculated.

In the final step of the analysis, this component (I) was combined with the two previously calculated components (II and III) into a matrix that was rotated by procedure of canonical matching towards the initial component matrix (A). The resulting matrix (B) is presented in table 13, in the text. The amount of variance explained by these three components is 65.3%. The similarity of matrix A and matrix B is large as shown by the congruence coefficients of .95, 1.0, and 1.0 for the first, second, and third components.

An alternative method of calculation leads to similar, though less clear-cut results. Table 25 presents a component matrix (C) that was computed directly from the matrix of partial

Table 25 *Tests: three principal components directly obtained from partial correlations (age constant) (Groups 4 and 5; N = 30)*

	dimension 1	dimension 2	dimension 3
Raven-matrices	.60	.19	.47
vocabulary	.83	–.22	–.29
arithmetic	.52	.60	–.02
Porteus-mazes	.22	.83	–.04
block-design	.24	.65	.33
memory-for-designs	.47	.32	.60
Knox-cubes	.68	.30	.65
learning	–.11	.67	.39
incidental-learning	–.18	–.05	.83

correlations (age constant) and rotated towards the initial component matrix (A), by procedure of canonical matching. The amount of variance explained by these three components is 66.0% (65.3% in the previous procedure). Although the pattern that emerges is less clear than that emerging from the matrices (A) and (B), mostly as regards the arithmetic, memory-for-designs, and learning tests, the overall pattern is nevertheless the same. Also the congruence coefficients for the first, second, and third factors of matrix (C) and matrix (A) are .88, .93, and .97. The agreement between the three components computed in this way and the three components calculated by the previous method is even higher. The congruence coefficients of the components 1,2, and 3 in matrix (C) and matrix (B) are 1.0, 1.0, and .82, respectively. The difference in results between the matrix (B) and the matrix (C) is caused by a slight reordering of the components. When all the possible (nine) components are calculated, canonical matching of matrix B and matrix C results in identical structures.

13. The objection may be raised that the particular type of analysis of variance used, a randomized block design, is not really appropriate in this case. This model of analysis assumes identical or near identical subjects in different conditions as, for example, when the same subjects are observed in different conditions or, as in agriculture, when a plot of land is divided into many small plots that are differently treated. Since the matching of different individuals is necessarily imperfect, it can be argued that these conditions are not met here. In that case, this particular analysis, because of its heightened sensitivity to differences, may perhaps have resulted in 'false positive' outcomes.

    To check on this, a one-way analysis of variance was also carried out for eight tests (excepting the memory-for-designs, see note 11), contrasting the three index groups with the group of comparison children. A one-way analysis of variance, although not really appropriate since the subjects in the different conditions were matched and not randomly selected, has at least the benefit of being less sensitive, with a reduced chance of 'false positive' outcomes. The results confirm those obtained with the previous, more sensitive, analysis. Block-design (p=.01), incidental learning (p=.01), and Lincoln-Oseretsky (chapter 7) (p=.02) are still significantly different, while vocabulary, arithmetic, Porteus-mazes, Knox-cubes, and learning are again not significantly different. The difference on the Raven-matrices, in the previous analysis, was just significant at the .05 level. The probability of this difference has now dropped to .08. Admittedly, this may shed some doubt on its meaning. There are, however, other indications that the scores on this test are affected by previous malnutrition, as will be shown later in this chapter.

14. Low correlations, such as found here, do not necessarily result from the absence of a relationship. In certain cases, such as with particular distributions of scores or nonlinear relations, a low correlation coefficient may nevertheless conceal a real relation. In the present study, however, there is no increase of test scores with age. For each child partial test scores were computed from which the contribution of education was removed. These partial test scores show no increase whatsoever with age when the mean scores for each test (except vocabulary) were computed for the five age groups into which the 60 index cases could be divided.
15. Richardson *et al.* (1973) have suggested that this absence of a relation with age may result from counteracting influences. Hospitalization retards development, but least in children younger than 6 months. The greater negative influence of hospitalization in older age groups might compensate for the greater impairment resulting from malnutrition at an early age. However, one important characteristic of malnutrition is the apathy of the children, and it seems unlikely that any further lack of stimulation could result from hospitalization. In the present investigation, moreover, most children were hospitalized for a short period of 2-3 weeks. Also, as is customary in Africa, the mother attended the child in the hospital, so that maternal deprivation was unlikely. Despite the fact that such 'compensation' seems unlikely in the present study, no differences were found between groups admitted at different ages.
16. See chapter 5 for a description of this last group.
17. These items are (22) throwing a ball at a target, (28) balancing on tiptoe, and (29) tapping with feet and fingers. There are no clear reasons why these particular items should be unsuitable among Baganda children. The possibility exists that the low item-total correlations of these items are chance variations resulting from the small number of children in this group.
18. The story that Edgerton tells of a father in Northern Kenya movingly illustrates this:

    'They [the Pokot] assert that while a man may do what he pleases with such "monsters" he actually ought to put them to death. A father in the Pokot tribe told me of the distress he felt in attempting to decide what to do about his daughter of 4, a profoundly retarded child unable to speak or control her bowels: "Two years ago I decided that she was useless. As you can see, she cannot do anything but sit there and eat dirt (feces) and laugh all the time. But when I took her to the river to drown her, she looked up at me and smiled and laughed. I couldn't do it then. So, I took her home and here she is." ' (Edgerton, 1970, p. 530.)

19. Individual scores are listed in appendix D.
20. With the exception of the behavioural ratings (chapter 8). On the very few occasions when it turned out to be extremely difficult to contact the parents for an interview, this was left to one of our interpreters, Mrs. Janet Kabanda.
21. One wonders also whether similar findings by Evans *et al.* (1971) which they attribute to differences in the social environment, are after all not genuine findings.

Appendices

Appendix A

Sex, age, and education of children in groups 1-4

Group 1. *Children admitted for protein-energy malnutrition between 8 and 15 months of age.*

Child, number	Sex	Age	Education
1	male	16.5	1.4
2	male	15.7	3.4
3	male	14.8	6.6
4	male	14.6	6.6
5	male	14.4	6.6
6	male	13.8	4.8
7	male	13.8	4.0
8	male	12.8	4.0
9	male	12.6	4.0
10	male	12.5	4.4
11	male	12.3	3.7
12	female	15.7	6.7
13	female	16.8	6.0
14	female	15.6	5.6
15	female	14.1	5.7
16	female	13.8	2.8
17	female	13.2	3.7
18	female	13.2	5.9
19	female	13.2	3.1
20	female	13.3	2.0

Group 2. *Children admitted for protein-energy malnutrition between 16 and 21 months of age.*

Child, number	Sex	Age	Education
21	male	15.8	4.0
22	male	14.3	4.7
23	male	16.4	6.4
24	male	14.0	5.7
25	male	13.8	4.8
26	male	12.8	5.2
27	male	13.4	3.7
28	male	12.8	4.1
29	male	12.5	4.4
30	male	11.7	4.4
31	male	13.8	2.8
32	female	16.3	7.0
33	female	16.8	5.0
34	female	16.6	4.0
35	female	13.3	5.6
36	female	13.8	3.0
37	female	13.3	3.8
38	female	13.4	5.9
39	female	13.3	3.4
40	female	12.8	2.0

Group 3. *Children admitted for protein-energy malnutrition between 22 and 27 months of age.*

Child, number	Sex	Age	Education
41	male	15.9	4.0
42	male	14.3	3.8
43	male	15.5	7.0
44	male	14.6	6.8
45	male	14.7	4.6
46	male	12.6	4.3
47	male	13.5	3.8
48	male	12.2	3.6
49	male	12.9	4.0
50	male	11.7	4.4
51	male	12.0	3.5
52	female	16.3	6.0
53	female	14.2	5.2
54	female	16.6	4.0
55	female	13.8	5.7
56	female	13.3	3.6
57	female	13.6	3.8
58	female	12.6	4.6
59	female	13.4	3.3
60	female	13.1	2.7

Group 4. *Comparison children.*

Child, number	Sex	Age	Education
61	male	14.0	3.3
62	male	14.8	4.6
63	male	16.0	7.6
64	male	15.7	6.0
65	male	15.7	5.4
66	male	13.4	4.8
67	male	12.6	3.4
68	male	12.8	4.0
69	male	12.8	4.2
70	male	11.8	5.5
71	male	12.5	1.5
72	female	16.7	6.0
73	female	15.6	5.6
74	female	15.7	5.0
75	female	13.3	5.0
76	female	12.8	3.3
77	female	13.2	3.9
78	female	13.2	4.0
79	female	12.8	2.6
80	female	11.8	2.7

Appendix B

Medical condition on admission of children in groups 1-3

Key:

I=	percentage of expected weight for age (Baganda standards).
II=	percentage of weight lost after admission.
III=	hæmoglobin (gm/100 ml).
IV=	serum protein (gm/100 ml).
V=	oedema rating (5= severe; 4= moderate; 3= slight; 2= trace; 1= none).
VI=	skin changes rating (4= severe; 3= moderate; 2= slight; 1= none).
VII=	overall clinical severity, rated by the attending doctor (5= severe; 4= poor; 3= moderate; 2= fair; 1= good).

Group 1. *Children admitted for protein-energy malnutrition between 8 and 15 months of age.*

Child, number	I	II	III	IV	V	VI	VII
1	64	15.0	6.3	2.9	4	4	5
2	57	1.7	2.6	4.4	4	3	4
3	64	5.5	8.4	5.8	4	4	4
4	79	0.0	10.0		2	2	2
5	78	12.4	9.4	4.7	3	2	2
6	79	3.2	5.2	3.5	3	2	2
7	73	17.5	2.8	3.1	4	4	5
8	77	10.1	7.6	5.1	3	1	2
9	66	5.0	6.2	4.6	4	1	4
10	89	22.0	7.7	3.3	5	4	4
11	82	7.3	6.7	4.2	4	4	3
12	71	2.1	7.8	4.7	4	2	4
13	50	6.4	6.3		3	2	2
14	53	0.6	4.5	5.8	3	3	3
15	56	0.0	7.7	5.5	2	1	2
16	59	13.6	7.0	4.0	4	3	4
17	58	0.0	2.8	4.4	3	3	4
18	56	2.0	9.7	4.7	2	2	3
19	63	7.6	7.4	3.3	3	4	4
20	67	3.1	3.1	3.7	5	1	4

Group 2. *Children admitted for protein-energy malnutrition between 16 and 21 months of age.*

Child, number	I	II	III	IV	V	VI	VII
21	72	12.5	9.2	4.7	4	2	3
22	86	1.5	7.0	3.7	4	3	3
23	85	2.3	9.1	4.0	4	4	3
24	72	8.6	7.0	3.5	4	4	3
25	76	11.0	8.8	4.7	4	1	3
26	68	22.5	7.9	3.3	5	4	4
27	80	8.9	7.0	3.7	4	2	2
28	63	12.2	6.7	2.9	4	3	4
29	71	18.4	3.4	4.7	4	3	3
30	89	10.3	8.6	4.1	3	2	2
31	42	1.0	5.5	3.3	3	2	3
32	79	9.5	10.5	5.1	4	2	2
33	64	3.0	9.0	5.0	2	2	4
34	68	6.6	7.7	4.5	2	4	4
35	65	3.8	4.2	5.1	4	1	3
36	55	6.1	3.9	4.4	5	3	5
37	59	25.2	7.6	4.4	5	3	5
38	64	8.2	5.3	5.1	3	2	2
39	70	10.6	4.0	3.8	4	3	4
40	68	2.9	5.8	5.1	3	3	3

Group 3. *Children admitted for protein-energy malnutrition between 22 and 27 months of age.*

Child, number	I	II	III	IV	V	VI	VII
41	66	7.8	9.2	3.6	4	4	5
42	80	14.7	6.9	4.0	5	4	3
43	76	10.4	8.7	4.2	4	2	3
44	64	8.6	8.3	3.7	4	2	3
45	71	6.3	5.6		4	2	2
46	85	13.7	9.0	5.1	4	3	4
47	73	0.0	2.8	4.2	4	3	3
48	64	7.2	6.8	3.9	3	3	3
49	75	3.1	7.4	4.7	4	4	4
50	70	11.6	7.3	3.6	4	4	3
51	63	12.5	7.5	4.1	4	4	3
52	66	4.3	6.6	4.0	3	1	2
53	74	4.2	3.5	3.3	5	3	3
54	79	17.4	6.9	4.2	4	2	4
55	71	10.8	7.4	3.7	5	3	4
56	68	3.8	7.4	4.7	4	4	4
57	76	6.8	5.0	4.0	4	1	2
58	75	15.8	3.6	2.9	4	4	4
59	78	16.8	9.0	4.0	4	3	2
60	72	8.2	7.9	3.9	4	3	3

Appendix C Test scores of children in groups 1-4

Group 1 *Children admitted for protein-energy malnutrition between 8 and 15 months of age.*

Child, number	Raven-matrices	vocabulary	arithmetic	Porteus-mazes	block-design	memory-for-designs	Knox-cubes	learning	incidental learning	Lincoln-Oseretsky
1	25	10	8	9	16	2	44	3	3	100
2	20	11	6	5	20	8	30	0	3	96
3	29	6	10	8	24	0	39	7	3	120
4	25	9	12	8	28	10	46	7	2	102
5	30	15	14	7	26	0	38	8	5	91
6	23	4	9	6	22	0	40	6	3	116
7	18	7	6	4	4	18	33	6	8	83
8	26	4	12	8	24	0	46	0	3	89
9	17	6	9	5	12	12	21	5	8	69
10	23	3	10	9	18	4	39	4	3	94
11	27	8	11	7	24	7	35	5	4	102
12	22	8	8	6	28	3	42	2	4	97
13	21	14	6	7	0	15	32	2	4	97
14	28	9	10	5	24	3	35	4	2	81
15	18	7	8	6	4	5	25	0	7	104
16	22	5	7	4	12	23	45	1	3	88
17	21	3	8	8	12	8	46	0	3	113
18	23	5	9	8	20	1	45	5	4	103
19	15	1	7	2	0	15	23	3	3	63
20	23	8	6	6	16	14	45	7	4	97

Group 2 *Children admitted for protein-energy malnutrition between 16 and 21 months of age.*

Child, number	Raven-matrices	vocabulary	arithmetic	Porteus-mazes	block-design	memory-for-designs	Knox-cubes	learning	incidental-learning	Lincoln-Oseretsky
21	23	14	12	7	18	8	41	1	4	108
22	24	13	11	7	22	0	34	8	5	87
23	31	14	13	8	22	5	47	3	6	106
24	26	7	11	8	16	5	36	7	3	8[illegible]
25	22	13	11	6	24	1	40	7	6	94
26	31	5	11	7	20	6	45	2	9	89
27	17	7	9	8	16	12	41	7	6	90
28	22	12	13	6	24	3	45	6	5	97
29	23	8	9	6	24	10	33	7	4	89
30	26	6	9	7	22	3	38	0	5	111
31	11	7	5	7	0	13	28	5	8	72
32	27	8	10	10	28	3	47	6	8	120
33	18	15	12	2	14	9	35	7	7	95
34	20	5	8	4	6	9	33	4	1	92
35	19	4	11	9	20	9	37	3	7	90
36	22	6	7	5	16	15	44	4	4	95
37	18	8	10	2	2	6	41	1	6	91
38	22	9	8	6	12	7	37	3	3	96
39	22	4	9	7	8	19	41	7	3	87
40	14	7	4	4	0	19	30	1	2	82

Group 3 *Children admitted for protein-energy malnutrition between 22 and 27 months of age.*

Child, number	Raven-matrices	vocabulary	arithmetic	Porteus-mazes	block-design	memory-for-designs	Knox-cubes	learning	incidental learning	Lincoln-Oseretsky
41	17	12	10	7	10	2	40	3	4	89
42	25	13	10	6	26	1	42	3	5	81
43	25	15	12	7	28	4	51	8	5	113
44	20	13	9	6	18	0	41	5	5	94
45	25	14	13	8	14	3	48	4	3	108
46	25	8	8	7	16	1	46	5	2	104
47	22	6	9	8	18	1	37	2	8	84
48	22	9	9	5	18	8	35	0	6	102
49	22	0	9	4	20	3	33	3	6	104
50	24	9	12	4	32	3	50	8	5	100
51	17	7	8	7	20	4	40	2	1	92
52	24	7	8	7	12	2	43	5	1	114
53	23	7	8	8	20	4	39	7	6	107
54	14	12	7	4	0	29	36	7	8	86
55	33	9	14	7	40	1	43	8	7	122
56	15	4	9	6	8	7	41	4	3	92
57	17	9	9	3	2	11	34	0	2	86
58	18	10	9	7	6	4	46	8	4	89
59	21	8	10	7	10	4	34	7	5	102
60	21	2	8	5	10	0	34	7	6	89

Group 4 *Comparison children.*

Child, number	Raven-matrices	vocabulary	arithmetic	Porteus-mazes	block-design	memory-for-designs	Knox-cubes	learning	incidental-learning	Lincoln-Oseretsky
61	20	7	8	8	24	4	38	6	8	121
62	22	7	9	8	26	10	42	7	5	103
63	34	19	12	10	24	4	47	8	5	124
64	25	18	11	9	32	0	41	4	7	116
65	27	6	15	9	28	0	45	8	7	94
66	24	7	7	8	22	18	27	6	6	70
67	21	10	11	6	12	12	27	1	2	99
68	27	2	6	7	32	0	40	5	8	115
69	17	14	8	8	14	5	33	2	4	119
70	27	7	12	7	24	0	38	8	4	120
71	18	5	8	7	20	7	35	0	3	104
72	27	9	8	6	16	0	42	8	6	113
73	28	15	12	7	24	8	32	8	7	103
74	27	18	6	2	8	13	33	0	4	117
75	24	5	11	6	24	2	41	8	8	116
76	24	10	7	8	24	1	52	1	9	91
77	22	2	8	8	20	9	48	8	5	74
78	22	10	8	4	20	3	40	4	8	95
79	22	2	7	6	24	9	48	4	4	101
80	24	6	11	6	20	0	42	6	7	81

Appendix D Behaviour ratings of children in groups 1-4

Group 1 *Children admitted for protein-energy malnutrition between 8 and 15 months of age.*

Child, number	household jobs	resting	slowness	activity	shyness	obedience	friendships
1	7	1	0	2	1	2	3
2	6	1	0	1	1	2	3
3	7	0	0	2	1	2	2
4	3	0	0	2	2	2	1
5	3	0	0	2	1	2	1
6	5	0	0	1	0	2	2
7	4	0	0	2	0	2	2
8	2	0	2	0	0	0	3
9	4	0	0	2	1	2	3
10	3	0	0	2	0	2	1
11	6	0	0	2	0	2	1
12	0	0	0	2	2	2	0
13	8						
14	4	1	2	1	0	2	0
15	5	0	1	2	1	2	2
16	6	1	0	2	2	2	0
17	6	1	0	2	0	2	3
18	3	0	0	1	0	2	3
19	2	1	0	2	0	2	3
20	6	0	0	2	1	2	0

Group 2 *Children admitted for protein-energy malnutrition between 16 and 21 months of age.*

Child, number	household jobs	resting	slowness	activity	shyness	obedience	friendships
21	3	1	0	1	2	1	2
22	3	0	0	1	0	1	1
23	3	1	0	2	0	2	2
24	5	0	0	2	1	2	2
25	2	0	0	2	1	2	1
26	2	1	0	1	0	2	3
27	3	0	2	1	0	2	3
28	2	1	0	1	1	2	3
29	2	1	0	1	1	0	3
30	4	0	2	2	2	2	2
31	0	1	2	0	0	2	2
32	5	0	0	1	0	2	1
33	4	1	1	0	0	2	2
34	8						
35	7	0	2	1	2	2	3
36	1	1	0	2	2	2	3
37	5	0	0	2	0	2	3
38	4	0	0	2	0	2	2
39	5	0	2	1	2	2	1
40	3	1	2	1	2	2	2

Group 3 *Children admitted for protein-energy malnutrition between 22 and 27 months of age.*

Child, number	household jobs	resting	slowness	activity	shyness	obedience	friendships
41	2	0	2	1	2	1	2
42	3	0	0	2	0	2	3
43	4	0	2	1	2	2	3
44	6	0	0	1	2	2	2
45	4	0	0	2	0	2	3
46	3	0	0	2	2	1	2
47	0	0	1	0	1	2	1
48	4	0	0	2	1	2	1
49	4	0	0	2	0	2	0
50	0	0	2	0	1	1	1
51	3	0	0	1	1	2	2
52	3	0	1	1	1	2	2
53	2	0	1	1	1	2	0
54	8						
55	5	1	0	2	2	2	0
56	5	0	0	2	1	2	2
57	3	0	1	2	2	2	3
58	4	1	0	1	1	2	2
59	3	0	0	2	0	2	2
60	4	1	0	2	0	2	2

Group 4 *Comparison children.*

Child, number	household jobs	resting	slowness	activity	shyness	obedience	friendships
61	1	1	2	0	2	1	2
62	0	0	0	0	1	0	3
63	2	0	0	1	1	2	0
64	6	0	0	2	0	2	2
65	1	0	0	2	2	0	2
66	1	0	0	2	1	1	2
67	5	0	0	2	0	2	2
68	7	0	0	2	0	2	3
69	4	0	0	2	2	2	2
70	4	0	2	2	2	2	3
71	0	0	0	2	0	2	3
72	1	0	1	0	0	1	1
73	1	0	0	2	0	2	2
74	8	1	1	1	1	2	0
75	2	0	0	1	0	1	0
76	6	0	2	1	0	2	2
77	0	0	0	1	1	2	1
78	7	0	0	2	0	1	1
79	3	0	2	1	2	2	2
80	2	0	0	2	1	2	1

Appendix E

Group 5: age, sex, education, test scores, and behaviour ratings

Child, number	Sex	Age	Education
81	male	16.3	7.5
82	male	14.9	6.7
83	male	14.3	6.6
84	male	12.6	1.0
85	male	12.3	5.4
86	male	11.5	3.4
87	female	16.5	6.7
88	female	15.2	7.0
89	female	15.0	7.0
90	female	13.8	5.3

Child, number	Raven-matrices	vocabulary	arithmetic	Porteus-mazes	block-design	memory-for designs	Knox-cubes	learning	incidental-learning	Lincoln-Oseretsky
81	28	12	13	9	24	1	41	8	5	115
82	21	13	12	7	16	10	38	4	4	92
83	33	11	13	9	28	2	48	6	8	128
84	21	9	12	8	16	4	47	7	5	78
85	25	11	12	8	28	2	35	8	4	102
86	23	2	10	7	32	0	46	7	9	74
87	29	14	14	8	18	6	44	8	9	118
88	33	18	15	8	32	3	43	5	3	98
89	26	12	11	5	6	6	44	8	10	101
90	25	0	8	4	16	6	31	4	6	91

Child, number	household jobs	resting	slowness	activity	shyness	obedience	friendships
81	0	0	0	1	0	0	2
82	4	0	0	2	0	2	3
83	2	0	0	1	1	2	3
84	1	1	0	2	0	0	3
85	3	0	0	2	2	2	3
86	3	0	0	2	0	0	3
87	5	0	0	2	1	2	2
88	4	1	0	1	0	2	1
89	8	0	0	2	1	2	3
90	3	0	0	0	2	2	3

Appendix F Arithmetic

(1) Count these [9] blocks with your finger.

(2) Take away all of the blocks except four, leave four blocks for yourself.

(3) Take away all the blocks except seven, leave seven blocks for yourself.

(4) If I cut an orange in half, how many pieces will I have?

(5) John had four shillings and his mother gave him two more. How many shillings did he have altogether?

(6) James had eight stones and he found six more. How many stones did he have altogether?

(7) A boy had twelve bananas and sold five of them. How many did he have left?

(8) One shirt costs seven shillings. How much will three shirts cost?

(9) A man had twenty-five cows and he sold eleven of them. How many did he have left?

(10) Four boys had seventy-two oranges. They divided them equally among themselves. How many oranges did each boy get?

(11) A workman earned thirty-six shillings. He was paid four shillings a day. How many days did he work?

(12) If you buy thirty tomatoes at twenty-five cents for ten, how many cents will they return to you from one shilling?

(13) Two-thirds of a number is 36. What is that number?

(14) If three pencils cost five cents, how much will twenty-four pencils cost?

(15) If a taxi charges twenty cents for the first mile and takes ten cents for every additional mile. How much money will be required to pay for a journey of eight miles?

Appendix G Socio-economic status

Percentage of families which pass each item (30 non-malnourished children; groups 4 and 5).

A. *'Modern Expenditure' scale*	
own table	70
condition of house, moderate or good	60
own radio	50
live in house with cement floor	47
own arm-chairs	27
own gramophone	17
own car	10
B. *'Traditional Resources' scale*	
live in house with 3 or more rooms	83
own bicycle	43
own 1 or more plots of farmland	37
own the plot of land on which their house is built	23
own 3 or more cows	13
employ 3 or more workers	7

References

Ainsworth, M. D. (1967). *Infancy in Uganda*. Baltimore: Johns Hopkins Press.

Anastasi, A. (1968). *Psychological testing* (3rd ed.). London: Macmillan.

Arthur, G. (1947). *A point scale of performance tests*. New York: Psychological Corporation.

Athayde, A. (1934). Tempos de reaccao de indigenas das colonias portuguesas. In *Trabalhos do 1. Congresso Nacional de Antropologia Colonial*, pp. 407-11. Porto.

Atlas of Uganda (2nd ed.) (1967). Uganda Government, Department of Land and Surveys.

Barg, B. (1973). Nutrition and national development. In A. Berg, N. S. Scrimshaw & D. L. Call (Eds.), *Nutrition, national development, and planning*, pp. 49-69. Cambridge, Mass.: M.I.T. Press.

Barker, D. J. P., & Bennett, F. J. (1973). *Practical epidemiology*. Edinburgh: Churchill Livingstone.

Bengoa, J. M. (1973). Significance of malnutrition and priorities for its prevention. In A. Berg, N. S. Scrimshaw & D. L. Call, *Nutrition, national development, and planning*, pp. 103-28. Cambridge, Mass.: M.I.T. Press.

Bennett, F. J., & Stanfield, J. P. (1971). The clinical conditions and aetiology of malnutrition in Uganda. *Journal of Tropical Pediatrics and Environmental Child Health*, 17, monograph 13, 5-10.

Berg, A. (1973). *The nutrition factor*. Washington: Brookings Institution.

Biesheuvel, S. (1952). Personnel selection tests for Africans. *South African Journal of Science*, 49, 3-12.

Biesheuvel, S. (1954). The measurement of occupational aptitudes in a multiracial society. *Occupational Psychology*, 28, 189-96.

Billewicz, W. Z. (1974a). Some remarks on cross-sectional and longitudinal studies in relation to malnutrition and its consequences. In *Symposia of the Swedish Nutrition Foundation XII, part 2,* pp. 49-56. Uppsala.

Billewicz, W. Z. (1974b). Some remarks on experimental intervention studies in relation to malnutrition and its consequences. In *Symposia of the Swedish Nutrition Foundation XII, part 2,* pp. 57-63. Uppsala.

Birch, H. G. (1972). Malnutrition, learning and intelligence. *American Journal of Public Health*, 62, 773-84.

Birch, H. G., Pineiro, C., Alcalde, E., Toca, T., & Cravioto, J. (1971). Relation of kwashiorkor in early childhood and intelligence at school age. *Pediatric Research*, 5, 579-85.

Botha-Antoun, E., Babayan, S., & Harfouche, J. K. (1968). Intellectual development related to nutritional status. *Journal of Tropical Pediatrics*, 14, 112-5.

Briers, P. J., Hoorweg, J., & Stanfield, J. P. (1975). The long term effects of protein energy malnutrition in early childhood on bone age, bone cortical thickness and height. *Acta Paediatrica Scandinavia*, 64, 853-8.

Brockman, L. M., & Ricciuti, H. N. (1971). Severe protein-calorie malnutrition and cognitive development in infancy and early childhood. *Developmental Psychology*, 4, 312-9.

Brown, R. E. (1966). Organ weight in malnutrition with special reference to brain weight. *Developmental Medicine and Child Neurology*, 8, 512-22.

Brown, R. E., & Opio, E. A. (1966). Associated factors in kwashiorkor in Uganda. *Tropical and Geographical Medicine*, 18, 119-24.

Brownlee, K. A. (1965). *Statistical theory and methodology in science and engineering*. New York: John Wiley.

Burgess, H. J. L. (1962a). Protein-calorie malnutrition in Uganda: Busoga district. *East African Medical Journal*, 39, 362-74.

Burgess, H. J. L. (1962b). Protein-calorie malnutrition in Uganda: Bukedi district. *East African Medical Journal*, 39, 375-85.

Burgess, H. J. L. (1962c). Protein-calorie malnutrition in Uganda: Bugisu district. *East African Medical Journal*, 39, 386-90.

Burgess, H. J. L. (1962d). Protein-calorie malnutrition in Uganda: Ankole district. *East African Medical Journal*, 39, 391-400.

Burgess, H. J. L. (1962e). Protein-calorie malnutrition in Uganda: Kigezi district. *East African Medical Journal*, 39, 401-10.

Burgess, H. J. L., & Burgess, A. P. (1972). Nutritional content and value of local foodstuffs: A critical appraisal. In V. F. Amann, D. G. R. Belshaw & J. P. Stanfield (Eds.), *Nutrition*

and food in an African economy, volume 1, pp. 45-58. Kampala: Makerere University, Department of Rural Economy.
Cabak, V., & Najdanvic, R. (1965). Effect of undernutrition in early life on physical and mental development. *Archives of Disease in Childhood*, 40, 532 4.
Campbell, D. T., & Stanley, J. C. (1966). *Experimental and quasi-experimental designs for research*. Chicago: Rand McNally.
Canosa, C. A. (1968). Ecological approach to the problems of malnutrition, learning, and behavior. In N. S. Scrimshaw & J. E. Gordon (Eds.), *Malnutrition, learning, and behavior*, pp. 389-96. Cambridge, Mass.: M.I.T. Press.
Champakam, S., Srikantia, S. G., & Gopalan, C. (1968). Kwashiorkor and mental development. *American Journal of Clinical Nutrition*, 21, 844-52.
Chase, H. P., & Martin, H. P. (1970). Undernutrition and child development. *New England Journal of Medicine*, 282, 933-9.
Chavez, A., Martinez, C., & Yaschine, T. (1974). The importance of nutrition and stimuli on child mental and social development. In *Symposia of the Swedish Nutrition Foundation XII, part 1*, pp. 211-25. Uppsala.
Cheek, D. B., Holt, A. B., & Mellits, E. D. (1972). Malnutrition and the nervous system. In Pan American Health Organization, *Nutrition, the nervous system, and behavior*, pp. 3-14. Washington.
Cleave, J. H. (1972). Food requirements and availability in Uganda: A national food balance sheet. In V. F. Amann, D. G. R. Belshaw & J. P. Stanfield (Eds.), *Nutrition and food in an African economy, volume 1*, pp. 109-25. Kampala: Makerere University, Department of Rural Economy.
Cole, M., Gay, J., Glick, J. A., & Sharp, D. W. (1971). *The cultural context of learning and thinking*. London: Methuen.
Cole, M., & Scribner, S. (1974). *Culture and thought: A psychological introduction*. New York: John Wiley.
Cravioto, J., Birch, H. G., DeLicardie, E., Rosales, L., & Vega, L. (1969). The ecology of growth and development in a Mexican preindustrial community. *Monographs of the Society for Research in Child Development*, 34, no. 5.
Cravioto, J., & DeLicardie, E. R. (1970). Mental performance in school age children. *American Journal of Diseases of Children*, 120, 404-10.
Cravioto, J., & DeLicardie, E. R. (1972). Environmental correlates of severe clinical malnutrition and language development in survivors from kwashiorkor or marasmus. In Pan American Health Organization, *Nutrition, the nervous system, and behavior*, pp. 73-94. Washington.
Cravioto, J., DeLicardie, E. R., & Birch, H. G. (1966). Nutrition,

growth and neurointegrative development: An experimental and ecologic study. *Pediatrics*, 38, 319-72.
Cravioto, J., & Robles, B. (1965). Evolution of adaptive and motor behaviour during rehabilitation from kwashiorkor. *American Journal of Orthopsychialry*, 35, 449-64.
Cryns, A. G. J. (1962). African intelligence: A critical survey of cross-cultural intelligence research in Africa South of the Sahara. *Journal of Social Psychology*, 57, 283-301.
Dasen, P. R. (1972). Cross-cultural Piagetian research: A summary. *Journal of Cross-cultural Psychology*, 3, 23-40.
Dean, R. F. A. (1954). Standards for African children and the influence of nutrition. *Journal of Tropical and Medical Hygiene*, 57, 283-9.
Dean, R. F. A., & Burgess, H. J. L. (1962). Protein-calorie malnutrition in Uganda: Conclusions of the survey and recommendations. *East African Medical Journal*, 39, 411-6.
DeLicardie, E. R., & Cravioto, J. (1974). Behavioral responsiveness of survivors of clinical severe malnutrition to cognitive demands. In *Symposia of the Swedish Nutrition Foundation XII, part 1*, pp. 134-53. Uppsala.
De Wet, D. R. (1967). An appraisal of sensory motor activities. *Psychologia Africana*, 12, 17-41.
Dobbing, J. (1968). Effects of experimental undernutrition on development of the nervous system. In N. S. Scrimshaw & J. E. Gordon (Eds.), *Malnutrition, learning, and behaviour*, pp. 181-202. Cambridge, Mass.: M.I.T. Press.
Dobbing, J. (1974). Prenatal development and neurological development. In *Symposia of the Swedish Nutrition Foundation XII, part 1*, pp. 96-110. Uppsala.
Dobbing, J., & Smart, J. L. (1974). Vulnerability of developing brain and behaviour. *British Medical Bulletin*, 30, 164-8.
Doll, R. (1959). Retrospective and prospective studies. In L.J. Witts (Ed.), *Medical surveys and clinical trials*, pp. 64-90. London: Oxford University Press.
Doob, L. W. (1965). Psychology. In R. Lystad (Ed.), *The African world: A survey of social research*, pp. 373-415. London: Pall Mall Press.
Dureman, I. (1974). Learning and perception: Psychophysiological aspects. In *Symposia of the Swedish Nutrition Foundation XII, part 2*, pp. 21-3. Uppsala.
Edgerton, R. B. (1970). Mental retardation in non-Western societies: Toward a cross-cultural perspective on incompetence. In H. C. Haywood (Ed.), *Social-cultural aspects of mental retardation*, pp. 523-59. New York: Appleton-Century-Crofts.
Edwards, L. D., & Craddock, L. J. (1973). Malnutrition and intel-

lectual development: A study in school-age aboriginal children at Walgett, N.S.W.. *Medical Journal of Australia*, 1, 880-4.

Evans, D. E., Moodie, A. D., & Hansen, J. D. L. (1971). Kwashiorkor and intellectual development. *South African Medical Journal*, 45, 1413-26.

Fallers, L. A. (1964). Social mobility, traditional and modern. In L. A. Fallers (Ed.), *The King's men: Leadership and status in Buganda on the eve of independence*, pp. 158-210. London: Oxford University Press.

Fallers, M. C. (1960). *The Eastern Lancustrine Bantu (Ganda, Soga)*. London: International African Institute.

Farmer, A. P. (1960). Malnutrition as an ecological problem. *East African Medical Journal*, 37, 399-404.

Faverge, J. M., & Falmagne, J. C. (1962). On the interpretation of data in intercultural psychology. *Psychologia Africana*, 9, 22-36.

Ferguson, G. A. (1951). A note on the Kuder-Richardson formula. *Educational and Psychological Measurement*, 11, 612-5.

Frankova, S. (1974). Interaction between early malnutrition and stimulation in animals. In *Symposia of the Swedish Nutrition Foundation XII, part 1*, pp. 202-9. Uppsala.

Frisch, R. E. (1970). Present status of the supposition that malnutrition causes permanent mental retardation. *American Journal of Clinical Nutrition*, 23, 189-95.

Frood, J. D. L., Whitehead, R. G., & Coward, W. A. (1971). Relationship between pattern of infection and development of hypoalbuminaemia and hypo-β-lipoproteinaemia in rural Ugandan children. *Lancet*, (2), 1047-9.

Gale, G. W. (1960). Food balance sheets for the African populations of East Africa. *East African Medical Journal*, 37, 410-7.

Geber, M., & Dean, R. F. A. (1956). The psychological changes accompanying kwashiorkor. *Courrier*, 6, 3-13.

Ghai, O. P., Ratna, K., Ramachandran, K., & Neki, J. S. (1973). Effect of early marasmic malnutrition on subsequent mental development. *Indian Pediatrics*, 10, 155-9.

Gongora, J., & McFie, J. (1959). Malnutrition, malaria and mortality: The use of a simple questionnaire in an epidemiological study. *Transactions of the Royal Society of Tropical Medicine and Hygiene*, 53, 238-47.

Graham, F. K., & Kendall, B. S. (1960). Memory-for-designs test: Revised general manual. *Perceptual and Motor Skills*, 11, 147-88.

Grant, G. V. (1970). Spatial thinking: A dimension in African intellect. *Psychologia Africana*, 13, 222-39.

Grant, G. V. (1972). The organization of intellectual abilities of an

African ethnic group in cultural transition. In L. J. Cronbach & P. J. D. Drenth (Eds.), *Mental tests and cultural adaptation*, pp. 391-400. The Hague: Mouton.

Grant, G. V. & Schepers, J. M. (1969). An exploratory factor analysis of five new cognitive tests for African mineworkers. *Psychologia Africana*, 12, 181-92.

Habicht, J-P., Martorell, R., Yarbrough, C., Malina, R. M., & Klein, R. E. (1974). Height and weight standards for preschool children: How relevant are ethnic differences in growth potential. *Lancet*, (1), 611-5.

Habicht, J-P., Yarbrough, C., & Klein, R. E. (1974). Assessing nutritional status in a field study of malnutrition and mental development. In *Symposia of the Swedish Nutrition Foundation XII, part 2*, pp. 35-42. Uppsala.

Hertzig, M. E., Birch, H. G., Richardson, S. A., & Tizard, J. (1972). Intellectual levels of school children severely malnourished during the first two years of life. *Pediatrics*, 49, 814-24.

Hoorweg, J., & Marais, H. C. (1969). *Psychology in Africa: A bibliography*. Leiden: African Studies Centre.

Hoorweg, J., & Stanfield, J. P. (1976). Protein-energy malnutrition of early childhood as it affects intellectual and motor abilities in the older child and adolescent. *Developmental Medicine and Child Neurology*, in press.

Horst, P. (1953). Correcting the Kuder-Richardson reliability for dispersion of item difficulties. *Psychological Bulletin*, 50, 371-4.

Irvine, S. H. (1969a). Factor analysis of African abilities and attainments: Constructs across cultures. *Psychological Bulletin*, 71, 20-32.

Irvine, S. H. (1969b). Figural tests of reasoning in Africa: Studies in the use of Raven's matrices across cultures. *International Journal of Psychology*, 4, 217-28.

Irvine, S. H. (1974). Contributions of ability and attainment testing in Africa to a general theory of intellect. In J. W. Berry & P. R. Dasen (Eds.), *Culture and cognition: Readings in cross-cultural psychology*, pp. 247-59. London: Methuen. (originally published in *Journal of Biosocial Science*, 1969, supplement 1, 91-102.)

Ishihara, S. (1959). *Tests for colour-blindness* (2nd ed.).' London: Lewis.

Jelliffe, D. B., Bennett, F. J., Stroud, C. E., Novotny, M. E., Karrach, H. A., Musoke, L. K., & Jelliffe, E. F. P. (1961). Field survey of the health of Bachiga children in the Kayonza district of Kigezi, Uganda. *American Journal of Tropical Medicine and Hygiene*, 10, 435-45.

Jelliffe, D. B., Bennett, F. J., White, R. H. R., Cullinan, T. R., & Jelliffe, E. F. P. (1962). The children of the Lugbara: A study in the techniques of paediatric field survey in tropical Africa. *Tropical and Geographical Medicine,* 14, 33-50.

Jelliffe, D. B., Bennett, F. J., Stroud, C. E., Welbourn ,H. F., Williams, M. C., & Jelliffe, E. F. P. (1963). The health of Acholi children. *Tropical and Geographical Medicine,* 15, 411-21.

Jelliffe, D. B., Bennett, F. J., Jelliffe, E. F. P., & White, R. H. R. (1964). Ecology of childhood disease in the Karamojong of Uganda. *Archives of Environmental Health,* 9, 25-36.

Jelliffe, D. B., & Stanfield, J. P. (1966). Protein deficiencies and calorie deficiencies. *Lancet,* (2), 907-8.

Kerlinger, F. (1973). *Foundations of behavioral research* (2nd ed.). London: Holt, Rinehart, and Winston.

Klein, R. E., Gilbert, O., Canosa, C., & De Leon, R. (1969). Performance of malnourished in comparison with adequately nourished children on selected cognitive tasks (Guatemala). Paper presented at the Annual Meeting of the American Association for the Advancement of Science; Boston, Mass; Dec. 30.

Klein, R. E., Habicht, J-P., & Yarbrough, C. (1971). Effects of protein-calorie malnutrition on mental development. *Advances in Pediatrics,* 18, 75-91.

Klein, R. E., Lester, B. M., Yarbrough, C., & Habicht, J-P. (1975). On malnutrition and mental development: Some preliminary findings. In A. Chavez, H. Bourges & S. Basta (Eds.), *Nutrition: Proceedings of the ninth international congress of nutrition, Mexico, 1972. Vol. 2,* pp. 315-21. Basel: Karger.

Klein, R. E., Yarbrough, C., Lasky, R. E., & Habicht, J-P. (1974). Correlations of mild to moderate protein-calorie malnutrition among rural Guatemalan infants and preschool children. In *Symposia of the Swedish Nutrition Foundation XII, part 1,* pp. 168-81. Uppsala.

Langlands, B. W. (1974). *Atlas of population census 1969 in Uganda.* Occasional paper no. 48. Kampala: Makerere University, Department of Geography.

Latham, M.C., & Cobos, F. (1971). The effects of malnutrition on intellectual development and learning. *American Journal of Public Health,* 61, 1307-24.

Levitsky, D. A., & Barnes, R. H. (1975). Malnutrition and the biology of experience. In A. Chavez, H. Bourges & S. Basta (Eds.), *Nutrition: Proceedings of the ninth international congress of nutrition, Mexico, 1972. Vol. 2,* pp. 330-4. Basel: Karger.

Liang, P. H., Hie, T. T., Jan, O. H., & Giok, L. T. (1967). Evaluation of mental development in relation to early malnutrition. *American Journal of Clinical Nutrition,* 20, 1290-4.

Lloyd, B. (1972). *Perception and cognition: A cross-cultural perspective.* Harmondsworth: Penguin.
Lloyd-Still, J. D., Hurwitz, I., Wolff, P. H., & Shwachman, H. (1974). Intellectual development after severe malnutrition in infancy. *Pediatrics*, 54, 306-11.
MacDonald, A. S. (1963). Some aspects of land utilization in Uganda. *East African Agricultural and Forestry Journal*, 29, 147-56.
Mair, L. (1934). *An African people in the twentieth century.* London: Routledge.
Marais, H. C., & Hoorweg, J. (1971). Psychology in Africa: A bibliographical survey. *International Journal of Psychology*, 6, 329-35.
May, J. M., & McLellan, D. L. (1970). *The ecology of malnutrition in Eastern Africa and four countries of Western Africa.* New York: Hafner.
McDowell, J. (1972). Patterns of protein availability and utilisation in Uganda. In V. F. Amann, D. G. R. Belshaw & J. P. Stanfield (Eds.), *Nutrition and food in an African economy, volume 1*, pp. 126-54. Kampala: Makerere University, Department of Rural Economy.
McLaren, D. S. (1974). The great protein fiasco. *Lancet*, (2), 93-6.
McLaren, D. S., Yaktin, U. S., Kanawati, A. A., Sabbagh, S., & Kadi, Z. (1973). The subsequent mental and physical development of rehabilitated marasmic infants. *Journal of Mental Deficiency Research*, 17, 273-81.
Mönckeberg, F. (1968). Effect of early marasmic malnutrition on subsequent physical and psychological development. In N. S. Scrimshaw & J. E. Gordon (Eds.), *Malnutrition, learning, and behavior*, pp. 181-202. Cambridge, Mass: M.I.T. Press.
Mönckeberg, F., Tisler, S., Toro, S., Gattas, V., & Vega, L. (1972). Malnutrition and mental development. *American Journal of Clinical Nutrition*, 25, 766-72.
Nesselroade, J. R., & Reese, H. W. (Eds.) (1973). *Life-span developmental psychology: Methodological issues.* New York: Academic Press.
Neuhäuser, G. (1975). Methods of assessing and recording motor skills and movement patterns. *Developmental Medicine and Child Neurology*, 17, 369-86.
Ombredane, A., Bertelson, P., & Beniest-Noirot, E. (1958). Speed and accuracy of performance of an African native population and of Belgian children on a paper-and-pencil task. *Journal of Social Psychology*, 47, 327-37.
Orley, J. H. (1970). *Culture and mental illness.* Nairobi: East African Publishing House.

Pollitt, E. (1972). Malnutrition, bio-social antecedents and cognitive development. *Revista de Neuro-Psiquiatria*, 35, 21-37. (*Psychological Abstracts*, 1973, 49, no. 6573).
Pollitt, E. (1973). Behavior of infant in causation of nutritional marasmus. *American Journal of Clinical Nutrition*, 26, 264-70.
Pollitt, E., & Granoff, D. (1967). Mental and motor development of Peruvian children treated for severe malnutrition. *Revista Interamericana de Psicologia*, 1, 93-102. (*Psychological Abstracts*, 1967, 41, no. 1169).
Porteus, S. D. (1937). *Primitive intelligence and environment*. New York: Macmillan.
Rao, K. S. J. (1974). Evolution of kwashiorkor and marasmus. *Lancet*, (1), 709-11.
Raven, J. C. (1965). *Guide to the coloured progressive matrices*. London: Lewis.
Richardson, S. A., Birch, H. G., Grabie, E., & Yoder, K. (1972). The behaviour of children in school who were severely malnourished in the first two years of life. *Journal of Health and Social Behaviour*, 13, 276-84.
Richardson, S. A., Birch, H. G., & Hertzig, M. E. (1973). School performance of children who were severely malnourished in infancy. *American Journal of Mental Deficiency*, 77, 623-32.
Riopelle, A. J. (1974). Early protein deprivation and behavioral deficit reconsidered. In *Symposia of the Swedish Nutrition Foundation XII, part 1*, pp. 127-33. Uppsala.
Roscoe, J. (1911). *The Baganda*. London: Macmillan.
Rutishauser, I. H. E. (1965). The heights and weights of middle class Baganda children. *Lancet*, (2), 565-7.
Rutishauser, I. H. E. (1971). Statistics of malnutrition in early childhood. *Journal of Tropical Pediatrics and Environmental Child Health*, 17, monograph 13, 11-6.
Rutishauser, I.H.E., & Whitehead, R.G. (1969). Field evaluation of two biochemical tests which may reflect nutritional status in three areas of Uganda. *British Journal of Nutrition*, 23, 1-13.
Rutishauser, I. H. E., & Whitehead, R. G. (1972). Energy intake and expenditure in 1-3 year old Ugandan children living in a rural environment. *British Journal of Nutrition*, 28, 145-52.
Sai, F. T. (1972). Nutrition as a priority in national development. In B. Vahlquist (Ed.), *Nutrition: A priority in African development*, pp. 137-48. Stockholm: Dag Hammarskjöld Foundation.
Savage, R. D. (1968). *Psychometric assessment of the individual child*. Harmondsworth: Penguin.
Savosnick, K. M. (1972). An economist's view of nutrition in its struggle for budgetary priority. In B. Vahlquist (Ed.), *Nutri-*

tion: A priority in African development, pp. 149-56. Stockholm: Dag Hammarskjöld Foundation.

Schaie, K. W. (1965). A general model for the study of developmental problems. *Psychological Bulletin*, 64, 92-107.

Schilling, F. (1970). Zur aussagefähigkeit des Oseretzkytests bei normalen und hirngeschädigten kindern. *Acta Paedopsychiatrica*, 37, 249-67.

Schneideman, I., Bennett, F. J., & Rutishauser, I. H. E. (1971). The nutrition rehabilitation unit at Mulago Hospital, Kampala: Development and evaluation, 1965-1967. *Journal of Tropical Pediatrics and Environmental Child Health*, 17, monograph 13, 25-34.

Scrimshaw, N. S., & Gordon, J. E. (Eds.) (1968). *Malnutrition, learning, and behavior*. Cambridge, Mass.: M.I.T. Press.

Sharman, A. (1972). Food consumption patterns in Eastern Uganda: A case study. In V. F. Amann, D. G. R. Belshaw & J. P. Stanfield (Eds.), *Nutrition and food in an African economy. volume 1*, pp. 70-94. Kampala: Makerere University, Department of Rural Economy.

Sloan, W. (1955). The Lincoln-Oseretsky motor development scale. *Genetic Psychology Monographs*, 51, 183-252.

Southwold, M. (1965). The Ganda of Uganda. In J. L. Gibbs (Ed.), *Peoples of Africa*, pp. 81-118. New York: Holt, Rinehart, and Winston.

Stanfield, J. P. (1972). Sequelae of malnutrition in early childhood. In V. F. Amann, D. G. R. Belshaw & J. P. Stanfield (Eds.), *Nutrition and food in an African economy, volume 1*, pp. 36-42. Kampala: Makerere University, Department of Rural Economy.

Stein, Z., Susser, M., Saenger, G., & Marolla, F. (1972). Intelligence test results of individuals exposed during gestation to the world war II famine in The Netherlands. *Tijdschrift voor Sociale Geneeskunde*, 50, 766-74.

Stewart, R. J. C. (1972). Small-for-dates offspring: An animal model. In Pan American Health Organization, *Nutrition, the nervous system, and behavior*, pp. 33-7. Washington.

Stewart, R. J. C., & Platt, B. S. (1968). Nervous system damage in experimental protein-calorie deficiency. In N. S. Scrimshaw & J. E. Gordon (Eds.), *Malnutrition, learning, and behavior*, pp. 168-80. Cambridge, Mass.: M.I.T. Press.

Stoch, M. B., & Smythe, P. M. (1967). The effect of undernutrition during infancy and subsequent brain growth and intellectual development. *South African Medical Journal*, 41, 1027-30.

Stuart, H. C., & Stevenson, S. S. (1954). Physical growth and development. In W. E. Nelson (Ed.), *Textbook of Paediatrics* (6th ed.), pp. 10-66. Philadelphia: Saunders.

Swedish Nutrition Foundation (1974). *Symposium XII; Part 1: Proceedings of a symposium on early malnutrition and mental development; Part 2: Workshop on methodology in studies of early malnutrition and mental development*, (Eds. J. Cravioto, L. Hambræus & B. Vahlquist). Uppsala: Almqvist and Wiksell.

Tizard, J. (1974a). Early malnutrition, growth and mental development in man. *British Medical Bulletin*, 30, 169-74.

Tizard, J. (1974b). Ecological studies of malnutrition: problems and methods. In *Symposia of the Swedish Nutrition Foundation XII, part 2*, pp. 64-71. Uppsala.

Truelove, S. C. (1959). Follow-up studies. In L. J. Witts (Ed.), *Medical surveys and clinical trials*. pp. 91-104. London: Oxford University Press.

Tuddenham, R. D. (1974). On analyzing longitudinal data relating nutrition to cognitive development. In *Symposia of the Swedish Nutrition Foundation XII, part 2*, pp. 72-82. Uppsala.

Turnbull, C. M. (1972). *The mountain people*. New York: Simon and Schuster.

Uganda Government (1972). *Third five-year development plan, 1971/2-1975/6.*

Valman, H. B. (1974). Intelligence after malnutrition caused by neonatal resection of ileum. *Lancet*, (1), 425-7.

Vandenberg, S. G. (1964). Factor analytic studies of the Lincoln Oseretsky test of motor proficiency. *Perceptual and Motor Skills*, 19, 23-41.

Vernon, P. E. (1969a). Abilities and educational attainments in an East African environment. In D. R. Price-Williams (Ed.), *Cross-cultural studies*, pp. 76-91. Harmondsworth: Penguin. (originally published in *Journal of Special Education*, 1967, 1, 335-45).

Vernon, P. E. (1969b). *Intelligence and cultural environment*. London: Methuen.

Vernon, P. E. (1971). *The structure of human abilities* (2nd ed.). London: Methuen. (originally published: 1950).

Wall, W. D., & Williams, H. L. (1970). *Longitudinal studies and the social sciences*. London: Heinemann.

Warren, N. (1970). Research design for investigation of the lasting behavioural effects of malnutrition: The problem of controls. *Social Science and Medicine*, 4, 589-93.

Warren, N. (1972). African Infant Precocity: A review of the evidence. *Psychological Bulletin*, 78, 353-67.

Warren, N. (1973). Malnutrition and mental development. *Psychological Bulletin*, 80, 324-8.

Waterlow, J. C., & Rutishauser, I. H. E. (1974). Malnutrition in man. In *Symposia of the Swedish Nutrition Foundation XII, part 1*, pp. 13-26. Uppsala.

Wechsler, D. (1949). *Wechsler Intelligence Scale for Children*. New York: Psychological Corporation.

Wechsler, D. (1955). *Wechsler Adult Intelligence Scale*. New York: Psychological Corporation.

Welbourn, H. F. (1955). The danger period during weaning. *Journal of Tropical Pediatrics*, (1), 34-46; (1), 98-111; (1), 161-73.

Welbourn, H. F. (1959). Backgrounds and follow-up of children with kwashiorkor. *Journal of Tropical Pediatrics*, 5, 84-95.

Welbourn, H. F. (1963). Custom and child health in Buganda: Methods of child rearing. *Tropical and Geographical Medicine*, 15, 124-33.

Werner, E. E., & Muralidharan, R. (1970). Nutrition, cognitive status and achievement motivation of New Delhi nursery school children. *Journal of Cross-cultural Psychology*, 1, 271-81.

Wharton, B. (1971). The mortality of malnutrition in early childhood in Uganda. *Journal of Tropical Pediatrics and Environmental Child Health*, 17, monograph 13, 17-24.

W. H. O. (1974). Malnutrition and mental development. *WHO Chronicle*, 28, 95-102.

Williams, C. D. (1935). Kwashiorkor, a nutritional disease of children associated with a maize diet. *Lancet*, (2), 1151-2.

Wilson, D. (1973). The economic analysis of malnutrition. In A. Berg., N. S. Scrimshaw & D. L. Call (Eds.), *Nutrition, national development, and planning*, pp. 129-44. Cambridge, Mass: M.I.T. Press.

Winer, B. J. (1971). *Statistical principles in experimental design* (2nd ed.). New York: McGraw-Hill.

Winick, M., Brasel, J. A., & Rosso, P. (1972). Some speculations on mechanisms involved in the effects of undernutrition on cellular growth. In Pan American Health Organization, *Nutrition, the nervous system, and behavior*, pp. 24-32. Washington.

Wober, M. (1969). The meaning and stability of Raven's matrices test among Africans. *International Journal of Psychology*, 4, 229-35.

Wober, M. (1974). Towards an understanding of the Kiganda concept of intelligence. In J.W. Berry & P.R. Dasen (Eds.), *Culture and cognition: Readings in cross-cultural psychology*, pp. 261-80. London: Methuen.

Zimmermann, R. R., Geist, C. R., Strobel, D. A., & Cleveland, T. J. (1974). Attention deficiencies in malnourished monkeys. In *Symposia of the Swedish Nutrition Foundation XII, part 1*, pp. 115-26. Uppsala.

ERRATA

page 67, table 15:
arithmetic, F = -0.03; read F = 0.03

page 72, table 17:
Raven-matrices, F = -1.10; read F = 1.10
Porteus-mazes, F = -0.14; read F = 0.14
block-design, F = -0.10; read F = 0.10

Erratum with Protein-Energy Malnutrition and Intellectual Abilities
(Jan Hoorweg)

Kolibri 360 GmbH
Ferdinand-Jühlke-Straße 7
99095 Erfurt, Deutschland
produktsicherheit@kolibri360.de